IBS ELIMINATION DIET COOKBOOK

The complete Guide to Finding Your FODMAP Triggers and Eating Well to Improve Your Gut Health

DR JANE T. RYAN

Copyright © 2023 by Dr Jane T. Ryan

INTRODUCTION

In the journey toward a healthier and more balanced life, we often find ourselves searching for the guiding light that will illuminate our path to wellness. Imagine embarking on a quest where the treasures you uncover aren't gold or jewels, but rather the radiant vitality that comes from within. This is the essence of the IBS Elimination Diet Cookbook – a compass that leads you through the intricate landscape of your body, offering you a chance to discover the incredible benefits of embracing a new way of nourishing yourself.

Just like a protagonist in a story, you hold the power to transform your narrative. The IBS Elimination Diet Cookbook isn't just a collection of recipes; it's a tool for empowerment. It empowers you to regain control over your digestive health, to understand the nuances of your body's responses to various foods, and to forge a deep connection between your mind and your plate.

As you flip through its pages, you'll find not just recipes, but anecdotes of courage and perseverance from those who have walked this path before you. These stories remind us that the road to wellness isn't always linear – it's a journey of self-discovery, a pilgrimage of patience, and a celebration of small victories.

Every ingredient you choose, every meal you prepare, becomes a brushstroke in the masterpiece of your well-being. The IBS Elimination Diet Cookbook whispers wisdom into your culinary choices, encouraging you to savor the symphony of flavors that resonate harmoniously with your body. It reminds you that this journey is not just about eliminating triggers, but about embracing nourishment that speaks to your soul.

With each meal, you step closer to liberation from the constraints of discomfort, making space for boundless energy, clear thoughts, and a radiant spirit. So, dear traveler on the road to wellness, let the IBS Elimination Diet Cookbook be your steadfast companion, your guide, and your source of inspiration. The path may be challenging, but it is paved with the promise of vitality, and every chapter turned brings you closer to a life that is truly, beautifully yours.

WHAT IS IBS

Irritable Bowel Syndrome (IBS) is a common gastrointestinal disorder characterized by a group of chronic symptoms that affect the large intestine, or colon. It is a functional disorder, meaning that it doesn't cause any structural damage to the intestines but can lead to significant discomfort and disruption in a person's daily life.

SYMPTOMS OF IBS:

1. Abdominal Pain or Discomfort: Individuals with IBS often experience abdominal pain or discomfort that can range from mild to severe Typically, this discomfort is alleviated after having a bowel movement.
2. Altered Bowel Habits:IBS can lead to changes in bowel movements, including diarrhea, constipation, or a combination of both. These changes are often accompanied by a sense of incomplete evacuation.
3. Bloating and Gas: Many IBS sufferers experience bloating and excessive gas, which can contribute to discomfort and a feeling of fullness.
4. Mucus in Stool: Some individuals notice the presence of mucus in their stool.
5. Changes in Stool Appearance: The appearance of the stool can change, varying from loose and watery to hard and lumpy.

TRIGGERS OF IBS:

While the exact cause of IBS remains unclear, there are several factors that are known to trigger or exacerbate its symptoms. These triggers can vary from person to person, and managing them is crucial in controlling the condition. Some common triggers include:

1. Dietary Factors: Certain foods can trigger IBS symptoms, including high-fat foods, spicy foods, caffeine, dairy products, artificial sweeteners, and foods high in gas-producing carbohydrates (FODMAPs).
2. Stress and Anxiety: Emotional stress and anxiety can lead to the exacerbation of IBS symptoms. The gut-brain connection plays a significant role in IBS, with stress affecting gut motility and sensitivity.
3. Gut Motility Issues: In IBS, the muscles of the intestines can contract excessively, leading to diarrhea, or too slowly, causing constipation.
4. Bacterial Overgrowth: An imbalance of gut bacteria, known as dysbiosis, can contribute to IBS symptoms. This can lead to increased gas production and changes in gut motility.
5. Hormonal Changes: Hormonal fluctuations, particularly in women, can influence bowel function. Many women with IBS report worsening symptoms during their menstrual periods.
6. Medications: Certain medications, such as antibiotics and some pain medications, can disrupt the balance of gut bacteria and trigger IBS symptoms.
7. Inflammation: Low-grade inflammation in the gut may contribute to IBS symptoms. The immune system's response to certain triggers could lead to increased gut sensitivity.

THE ADVANTAGES OF AN ELIMINATION DIET FOR IBS

1. Identification of Trigger Foods: One of the primary advantages of an elimination diet is its ability to help individual pinpoint specific foods that trigger their IBS symptoms. By temporarily removing certain foods known to cause irritation, participants can observe how their body responds and determine which items are problematic.

2. Symptom Relief: IBS sufferers often experience a wide range of symptoms, from diarrhea to constipation and abdominal pain. Through the elimination diet, individuals can experience relief from these symptoms by avoiding foods that aggravate their condition.

3. Personalized Approach: Each person's triggers can vary widely, making it essential to personalize their dietary choices. An elimination diet empowers individuals to discover their unique trigger foods, allowing them to tailor their eating habits accordingly.

4. Enhanced Quality of Life: The chronic nature of IBS can have a negative impact on daily life and well-being. With symptom reduction through the elimination diet, individuals may experience an improved quality of life, better sleep, and increased overall comfort.

5. Scientifically-Guided Approach: While it's a self-guided process, an elimination diet is best undertaken with the guidance of a healthcare professional. Dietitians or doctors can help individuals create a strategic plan, ensure nutritional adequacy, and monitor progress throughout the process.

6. Learning Dietary Tolerance: As participants reintroduce eliminated foods one at a time, they can gauge their tolerance levels and identify specific thresholds for each trigger food. This knowledge empowers them to make informed decisions about their diet in the long run.

7. Reduced Dependence on Medication: While medication can provide temporary relief, an elimination diet tackles the root cause by addressing dietary triggers. This can potentially lead to a decreased reliance on medications to manage IBS symptoms.

8. Encourages Mindful Eating: The elimination diet requires individuals to pay close attention to what they eat and how their bodies react. This heightened awareness promotes mindful eating habits, fostering a better connection between food choices and overall well-being.

9. Long-Term Management Strategy: Once trigger foods are identified, individuals can establish a long-term dietary strategy that minimizes symptom flare-ups. This sustainable approach can help prevent IBS symptoms from disrupting daily life.

10. Sense of Empowerment: IBS can be frustrating and unpredictable, but successfully navigating an elimination diet can instill a sense of empowerment and control over one's health. It encourages individuals to actively participate in managing their condition.

1

BREAKFASTS

QUINOA PORRIDGE WITH BERRIES

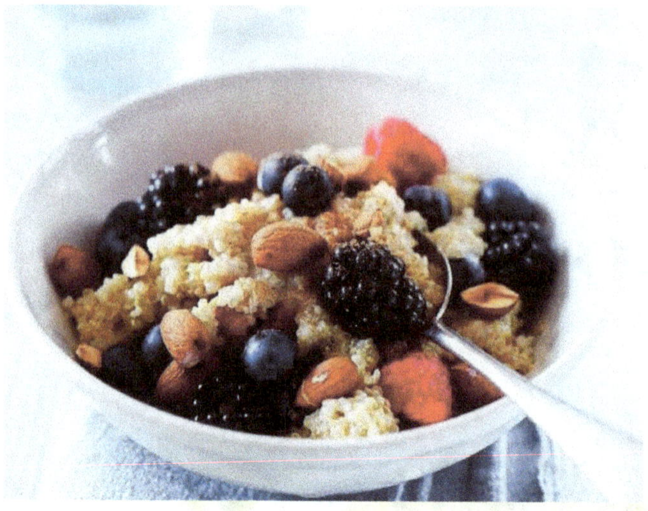

INGREDIENTS:

- 1/2 cup quinoa, rinsed
- 1 cup water or low-FODMAP vegetable broth
- 1 cup lactose-free almond milk or other tolerated non-dairy milk
- 1/2 cup mixed berries (blueberries, strawberries, raspberries)
- 1 tablespoon chia seeds
- 1 tablespoon maple syrup (optional, for sweetness)
- 1/2 teaspoon ground cinnamon
- A pinch of salt

PROCEDURE:

- Rinse the quinoa in a fine-mesh strainer with cold water to get rid of any bitter taste.
- In a medium saucepan, combine the rinsed quinoa, water or low-FODMAP vegetable broth, and a pinch of salt.
- Bring the mixture to a boil, then reduce the heat to low, cover the pot, and let it simmer for around 15 minutes until the liquid is absorbed.
- Once the quinoa is cooked, add the lactose-free almond milk, chia seeds, ground cinnamon, and maple syrup (if using). Stir well and continue to cook for another 5-7 minutes until the mixture thickens.
- Remove the saucepan from the heat and let the porridge sit for a few minutes to cool slightly.
- Transfer the quinoa porridge to serving bowls and top with a generous handful of mixed berries.
- Garnish with an extra sprinkle of cinnamon or chia seeds if desired.

NUTRITIONAL VALUE (PER SERVING):

- Calories: ~300
- Carbohydrates: ~50g
- Fiber: ~8g
- Protein: ~7g
- Fat: ~7g
- Vitamin C: ~30% of daily recommended intake
- Iron: ~15% of daily recommended intake
- Calcium: ~25% of daily recommended intake

HEALTH BENEFITS:

- Soluble Fiber Content: Quinoa is an excellent source of soluble fiber, which can aid in reducing IBS symptoms like bloating and diarrhea. It also supports overall gut health by promoting the growth of beneficial gut bacteria.
- Low-FODMAP Ingredients: This recipe features low-FODMAP ingredients like quinoa, lactose-free almond milk, berries, and chia seeds, making it suitable for individuals with IBS who are following the elimination phase.
- Antioxidant-Rich Berries: Berries are packed with antioxidants that help reduce inflammation and oxidative stress in the gut, potentially alleviating IBS symptoms.
- Chia Seeds: Chia seeds are an excellent source of soluble fiber and omega-3 fatty acids. They can contribute to a feeling of fullness and aid in regulating bowel movements.
- Cinnamon: Cinnamon possesses anti-inflammatory properties and may help soothe gastrointestinal discomfort often experienced by individuals with IBS.
- Nutrient Density: This porridge provides essential vitamins and minerals such as vitamin C, iron, and calcium, which are important for overall well-being and energy levels.

SCRAMBLED TOFU BREAKFAST TACOS

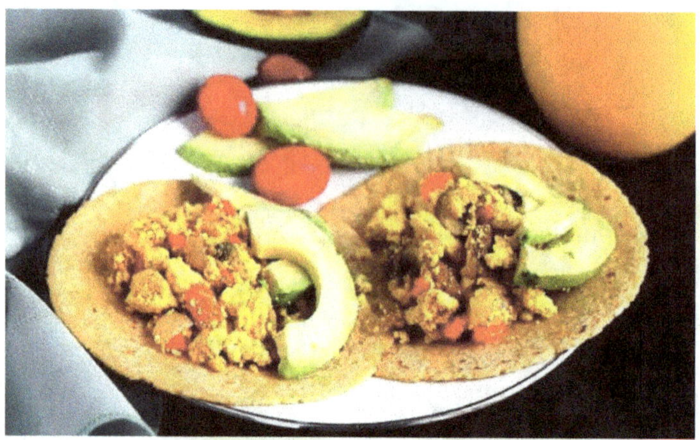

INGREDIENTS:

- 1/2 block firm tofu, drained and crumbled
- 1 tablespoon garlic-infused olive oil
- Try adding a mix of diced bell peppers in your dish - red, yellow, or orange - about half a cup.
- 1/4 cup diced scallions (green parts only)
- 1/4 teaspoon turmeric powder
- 1/4 teaspoon paprika
- Salt and pepper to taste
- 2-3 small corn tortillas (gluten-free)
- 1/4 avocado, sliced
- Fresh cilantro leaves for garnish
- Lactose-free or dairy-free yogurt (optional, for topping)

PROCEDURE:

- Warm the garlic-infused olive oil in a pan over medium heat.
- Add the diced bell peppers and sauté until they start to soften, about 2-3 minutes.
- Incorporate the diced scallions and continue cooking for an additional 1-2 minutes.
- Add the crumbled tofu to the skillet.
- Mix the tofu with turmeric, paprika, salt, and pepper. Stir gently to make sure the spices are evenly distributed.
- Heat the tofu mixture for 5-7 minutes, stirring it every now and then. The tofu should take on a golden hue from the turmeric.
- While the tofu cooks, warm the corn tortillas on a dry skillet or in the microwave.
- Once the tofu is cooked and heated through, remove the skillet from the heat.

- **Assembling the Tacos:**
- Place a spoonful of the scrambled tofu onto each warmed corn tortilla.
- Top with slices of avocado for creaminess and extra nutrition.
- For an extra burst of flavor and a pop of color, top off your dish with some fresh cilantro leaves.
- If desired, add a dollop of lactose-free or dairy-free yogurt for a tangy kick.

NUTRITIONAL VALUE (PER SERVING, 2 TACOS):

- Calories: ~250
- Carbohydrates: ~20g
- Fiber: ~4g
- Protein: ~12g
- Fat: ~15g
- Vitamin A: ~40% of daily recommended intake
- Vitamin C: ~70% of daily recommended intake
- Calcium: ~20% of daily recommended intake
- Iron: ~15% of daily recommended intake

HEALTH BENEFITS:

- Plant-Based Protein: Tofu is a valuable plant-based protein source that can be easier to digest
- than animal proteins for individuals with IBS. It's low in FODMAPs and supports muscle health.
- Turmeric: Turmeric's active compound, curcumin, has anti-inflammatory properties that can aid in reducing gut inflammation and IBS symptoms.
- Low-FODMAP Ingredients: This recipe features low-FODMAP veggies like bell peppers and scallions, making it suitable for IBS elimination phase.
- Avocado: Avocado's healthy fats and fiber content contribute to feelings of fullness, making it an excellent choice for individuals with IBS who may experience appetite fluctuations.
- Cilantro: Cilantro is known for its potential to support digestion and alleviate digestive discomfort, common in IBS.
- Nutrient Density: These tacos provide essential vitamins and minerals, including vitamin A, vitamin C, calcium, and iron, contributing to overall well-being.

BANANA OAT PANCAKES

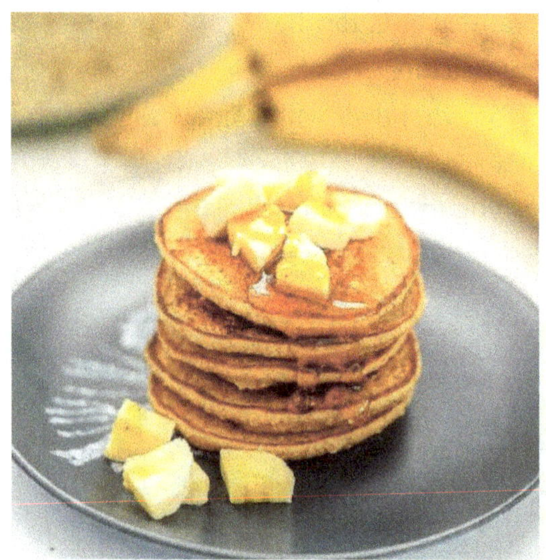

INGREDIENTS:

- 1 ripe banana, mashed
- 1 cup gluten-free rolled oats
- 2 large eggs
- 1/4 cup lactose-free or non-dairy milk (such as almond or rice milk)
- 1/2 teaspoon vanilla extract
- 1/2 teaspoon ground cinnamon
- 1/4 teaspoon baking powder
- Pinch of salt
- For the pan, you can use either coconut oil or a cooking spray.

PROCEDURE:

- In a blender or food processor, combine the mashed banana, gluten-free rolled oats, eggs, lactose-free or non-dairy milk, vanilla extract, ground cinnamon, baking powder, and a pinch of salt.
- Mix until everything is blended together and evenly distributed. If the batter appears too thick, you can add a little more milk to achieve the desired consistency.
- Let the batter sit for around 10 minutes. This helps the oats absorb the liquids and thicken the batter.
- Heat up a non-stick pan or griddle on medium heat. Lightly grease the surface with coconut oil or cooking spray.
- Once the skillet is heated, pour a small amount of batter onto the skillet to form pancakes of your desired size.

- Fry the pancakes for 2-3 minutes on one side, until you notice little bubbles appearing on the top.
- Gently flip the pancakes and cook for an additional 2-3 minutes on the other side, until they are golden brown and cooked through.
- Continue this process until all the batter has been used, adjusting the heat as needed to prevent burning.

NUTRITIONAL VALUE (PER SERVING, 3 PANCAKES):

- Calories: ~300
- Carbohydrates: ~45g
- Fiber: ~6g
- Protein: ~10g
- Fat: ~9g
- Vitamin B6: ~15% of daily recommended intake
- Magnesium: ~20% of daily recommended intake
- Potassium: ~10% of daily recommended intake

HEALTH BENEFITS:

- Low-FODMAP: This recipe uses low-FODMAP ingredients like ripe bananas, gluten-free rolled oats, and lactose-free or non-dairy milk, making it suitable for individuals with IBS during the elimination phase.
- Oats: Rolled oats are a good source of soluble fiber, which can help regulate bowel movements and ease digestive discomfort often experienced by individuals with IBS.
- Bananas: Ripe bananas are rich in potassium and easily digestible carbohydrates, making them a gentle option for those with sensitive digestive systems.
- Eggs: Eggs provide high-quality protein and essential nutrients that support muscle health and overall well-being.
- Cinnamon: Cinnamon possesses anti-inflammatory properties and can help soothe gastrointestinal irritation often associated with IBS.
- Vitamins and Minerals: This recipe contributes to daily nutrient intake, including vitamin B6, magnesium, and potassium, which are important for nerve function and muscle health.

2

SOUPS AND SALADS

GUT-HEALING BONE BROTH SOUP

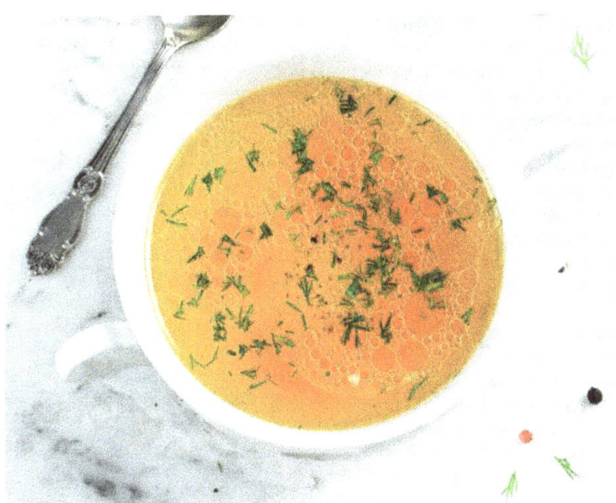

INGREDIENTS:

- **For the Bone Broth:**
- 2-3 pounds of grass-fed beef bones or organic chicken bones
- 2 carrots, roughly chopped
- 2 celery stalks, roughly chopped
- 1 onion, roughly chopped
- 3-4 cloves of garlic, crushed
- 1 tablespoon apple cider vinegar
- 1 teaspoon whole black peppercorns
- 1 bay leaf
- Filtered water
- **For the Soup:**
- 2 cups of bone broth
- 1 cup cooked and shredded chicken or beef (from the bones used for the broth)
- 1 cup chopped carrots
- 1 cup chopped zucchini
- 1 cup chopped spinach or kale
- Salt and pepper to taste
- Freshly chopped herbs (such as parsley or thyme) for garnish

PROCEDURE:

1. **Preparing the Bone Broth:**
   - Roast the bones in the oven at 400°F (200°C) for about 30 minutes to enhance the flavor.

- Place the roasted bones in a large stockpot along with chopped carrots, celery, onion, garlic, black peppercorns, bay leaf, and apple cider vinegar.
- Cover the ingredients with filtered water, ensuring they are fully submerged.
- Bring the pot to a boil, then reduce the heat to a low simmer.
- Allow the broth to simmer for at least 12-24 hours.
- Skim off any foam or other substances that come to the top. Once done, strain the broth into a container and discard the solids. Allow it to cool before refrigerating.

2. **Making the Gut-Healing Bone Broth Soup:**
   - In a separate pot, warm 2 cups of the prepared bone broth.
   - Add in the chopped carrots and zucchini. Simmer until they are tender.
   - Add the cooked and shredded chicken or beef to the pot.
   - Stir in the chopped spinach or kale and let them wilt.
   - Season the soup with salt and pepper according to taste.

3. **Serving:**
   - Ladle the warm gut-healing bone broth soup into bowls. Garnish with freshly chopped herbs, such as parsley or thyme, for added flavor and visual appeal.

NUTRITIONAL VALUE (PER SERVING):

- Calories: Approximately 150-200 kcal
- Protein: 15-20g
- Carbohydrates: 10-15g
- Fat: 5-7g
- Fiber: 2-3g

HEALTH BENEFITS:

- Gut Health: Bone broth is rich in collagen and gelatin, which are soothing for the digestive tract and can aid in repairing the gut lining.
- Anti-Inflammatory: The amino acids present in bone broth have anti-inflammatory properties, which can help reduce inflammation in the gut.
- Nutrient-Rich: Bone broth is a source of various nutrients like vitamins, minerals, and amino acids that support overall health.
- Easy Digestion: The gentle cooking process of bone broth makes it easy to digest, making it suitable for individuals with sensitive stomachs.
- Immune Support: The nutrients in bone broth can contribute to a healthy immune system, important for those with IBS.

MIXED GREENS WITH GRILLED CHICKEN AND LEMON-TAHINI DRESSING

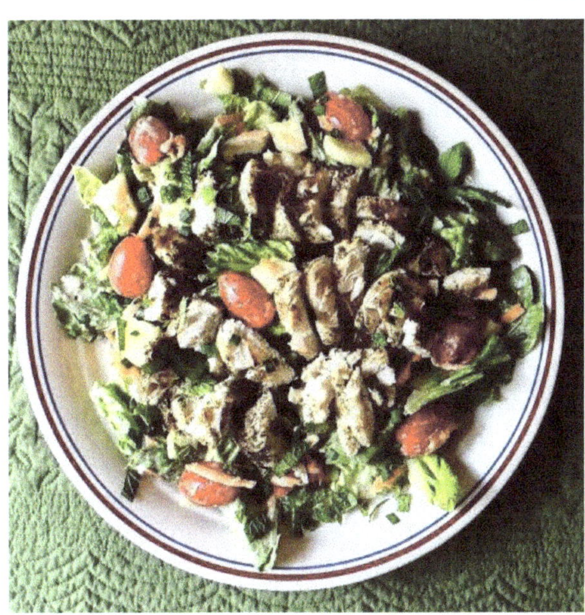

INGREDIENTS:

- **For the Salad:**
- 2 boneless, skinless chicken breasts
- 6 cups mixed greens (such as spinach, arugula, and butter lettuce)
- 1 cup cucumber, sliced
- 1 cup cherry tomatoes, halved
- 1/2 cup shredded carrots
- 1/4 cup sliced red onion
- Try adding a quarter cup of freshly chopped herbs like parsley, mint, or basil to your dish.
- Salt and pepper to taste
- **For the Lemon-Tahini Dressing:**
- 3 tablespoons tahini
- 3 tablespoons fresh lemon juice
- 2 tablespoons water
- 1 tablespoon extra-virgin olive oil
- 1 clove garlic, minced
- Salt and pepper to taste

PROCEDURE:

1. **Grilling the Chicken:**
   - Preheat a grill or grill pan over medium-high heat.

- Season the chicken breasts with salt and pepper on both sides.
- Grill the chicken for about 6-7 minutes on each side, or until the internal temperature reaches 165°F (74°C) and the chicken is no longer pink in the center.
- Remove the chicken from the grill and let it rest for a few minutes before slicing.

2. **Preparing the Lemon-Tahini Dressing:**
   - In a bowl, whisk together the tahini, fresh lemon juice, water, extra-virgin olive oil, minced garlic, salt, and pepper.
   - Adjust the consistency by adding more water if needed.
   - The dressing should be creamy and able to be poured.

3. **Assembling the Salad:**
   - In a large bowl, combine the mixed greens, sliced cucumber, halved cherry tomatoes, shredded carrots, sliced red onion, and chopped fresh herbs.
   - Toss the salad ingredients gently to combine.

4. **Adding Grilled Chicken:**
   - Arrange the sliced grilled chicken on top of the mixed greens.

5. **Dressing the Salad:**
   - Drizzle the lemon-tahini dressing over the salad according to your taste preferences.
   - Toss the salad gently to coat the ingredients with the dressing.

6. **Serving:**
   - Portion the mixed greens with grilled chicken and lemon-tahini dressing onto serving plates.
   - If you'd like, you can add some extra salt and pepper to taste.

NUTRITIONAL VALUE (PER SERVING):

- Calories: Approximately 300-350 kcal
- Protein: 25-30g
- Carbohydrates: 15-20g
- Fat: 15-18g
- Fiber: 4-6g

HEALTH BENEFITS:

- Lean Protein: Grilled chicken provides lean protein that's easy on the digestive system and supports muscle health.
- Fiber-Rich Greens: Mixed greens offer dietary fiber, aiding digestion and promoting a healthy gut environment.
- Anti-Inflammatory: Fresh herbs and olive oil in the dressing contain anti-inflammatory compounds that can alleviate IBS-related discomfort.

- Tummy-Friendly Dressing: Tahini is a creamy and tummy-friendly base for the dressing, while lemon juice adds a burst of flavor without triggering symptoms.
- Vitamins and Minerals: The salad is rich in vitamins A, C, K, and various minerals, supporting overall health and immunity.

ROASTED VEGETABLE SALAD WITH LEMON-HERB VINAIGRETTE

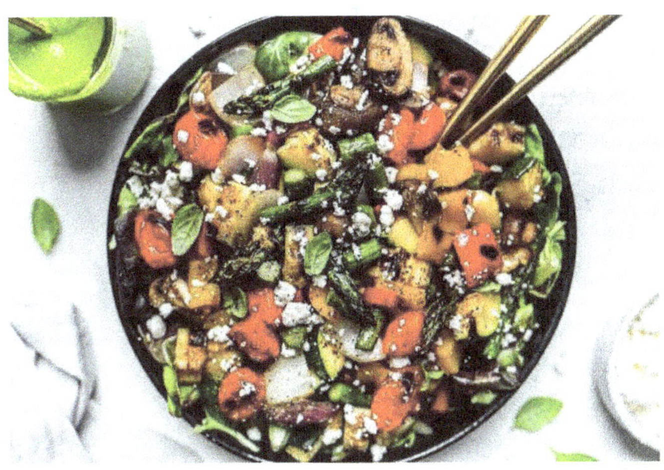

INGREDIENTS:

- **For the Salad:**
- 2 cups mixed vegetables (such as bell peppers, zucchini, carrots, and eggplant), cut into bite-sized pieces
- 1 cup cherry tomatoes, halved
- 1 cup baby spinach or mixed greens
- 1/4 cup red onion, thinly sliced
- 2 tablespoons olive oil
- Salt and pepper to taste
- For the Lemon-Herb Vinaigrette:
- 3 tablespoons extra-virgin olive oil
- 2 tablespoons fresh lemon juice
- 1 teaspoon Dijon mustard
- 1 tablespoon fresh herbs (such as basil, parsley, or thyme), finely chopped
- 1 clove garlic, minced
- Salt and pepper to taste

PROCEDURE:

1. **Roasting the Vegetables:**
   - Preheat the oven to 400°F (200°C).
   - In a bowl, toss the mixed vegetables with olive oil, salt, and pepper until well coated.

- Arrange the vegetables on a baking sheet in a single layer.
- Roast the vegetables in the preheated oven for about 20-25 minutes, or until they are tender and slightly caramelized. Stir the vegetables halfway through the cooking time.
- Once roasted, remove the vegetables from the oven and let them cool slightly.

2. **Preparing the Lemon-Herb Vinaigrette:**
   - In a small bowl, whisk together the extra-virgin olive oil, fresh lemon juice, Dijon mustard, chopped herbs, minced garlic, salt, and pepper.
   - Adjust the seasoning and acidity according to your taste preferences.

3. **Assembling the Salad:**
   - In a large salad bowl, combine the roasted vegetables, halved cherry tomatoes, baby spinach or mixed greens, and thinly sliced red onion.
   - Toss the salad ingredients gently to distribute the flavors.

4. **Dressing the Salad:**
   - Drizzle the lemon-herb vinaigrette over the salad according to your preference.
   - Toss the salad gently to coat the ingredients with the dressing.

5. **Serving:**
   - Portion the dressed roasted vegetable salad onto serving plates.
   - If you'd like, you can add some extra salt and pepper to taste.

NUTRITIONAL VALUE (PER SERVING):

- Calories: Approximately 180-220 kcal
- Protein: 2-3g
- Carbohydrates: 10-15g
- Fat: 15-18g
- Fiber: 4-6g

HEALTH BENEFITS:

Fiber-Rich Vegetables: Roasted vegetables offer dietary fiber, aiding digestion and promoting gut health in individuals with IBS.

Low-FODMAP Option: Many roasted vegetables used in this recipe are low in fermentable carbohydrates, making it suitable for those following a low-FODMAP diet for IBS.

Vitamin and Mineral Boost: The assortment of colorful vegetables provides essential vitamins, minerals, and antioxidants for overall well-being.

Gentle on Digestion: Roasting vegetables can break down some of the fibers, making them easier to digest while retaining nutritional value.

Digestive Comfort: The lemon-herb vinaigrette adds zest and flavor without triggering IBS symptoms, enhancing the eating experience.

3

MAIN DISHES: VEGETARIAN

ZUCCHINI NOODLES WITH PESTO AND CHERRY TOMATOES

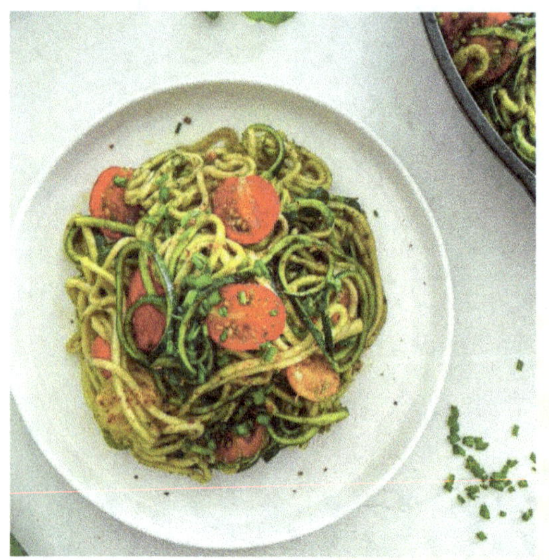

INGREDIENTS:

- 2 medium zucchinis
- 1 cup cherry tomatoes, halved
- 1/4 cup pine nuts (or walnuts for a low-FODMAP option)
- 2 cups fresh basil leaves
- 1/2 cup grated Parmesan cheese (omit for a dairy-free version)
- 1/2 cup olive oil
- 2 cloves garlic (use garlic-infused oil for a low-FODMAP option)
- Salt and pepper to taste
- 1 tablespoon lemon juice
- 1 tablespoon grated lemon zest
- Fresh basil leaves for garnish

PROCEDURE:

1. **Zucchini Noodles:**
   - Wash and trim the ends of the zucchinis. Use a spiralizer to create zucchini noodles.
   - Place the zucchini noodles in a colander, sprinkle with salt, and let them sit for about 15-20 minutes to release excess moisture.
   - Rinse the noodles thoroughly and pat them dry with a clean kitchen towel.
2. **Pesto:**
   - In a dry skillet, lightly toast the pine nuts until they are fragrant and golden. Let them cool.
   - In a food processor, combine the basil leaves, toasted pine nuts, Parmesan cheese (if using), garlic, lemon juice, and lemon zest.

- Pulse the mixture while gradually adding the olive oil until the pesto reaches your desired consistency.
- Season with salt and pepper to taste.

3. **Assembly:**
   - In a large mixing bowl, gently toss the zucchini noodles with the homemade pesto until they are well coated.
   - Mix in the cut cherry tomatoes and give everything another stir.
   - Divide the zucchini noodle mixture into serving plates.
   - Top off your dish with some fresh basil leaves and a sprinkle of extra Parmesan cheese, if you like.

NUTRITIONAL VALUE (PER SERVING):

- Note:The nutritional content of a dish can vary depending on the portion size and ingredients used.
- Calories: 350 kcal
- Carbohydrates: 10g
- Protein: 8g
- Fat: 32g
- Fiber: 3g

HEALTH BENEFITS:

- Low FODMAP: This recipe follows the principles of the low FODMAP diet, which can help manage symptoms of IBS by reducing fermentable carbohydrates that can trigger discomfort.
- Zucchini: Rich in water and fiber, zucchini is gentle on the digestive system and helps maintain bowel regularity.
- Tomatoes: Cherry tomatoes provide vitamins A and C, and their natural acidity can aid digestion.
- Basil: This herb has anti-inflammatory properties and may soothe digestive issues.
- Pine Nuts: A source of healthy fats and protein, pine nuts are also rich in magnesium, which can support muscle relaxation and bowel function.

LENTIL AND SWEET POTATO CURRY

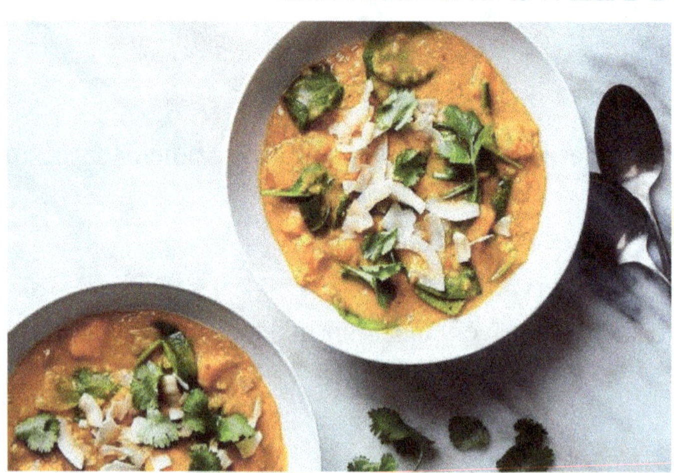

INGREDIENTS:

- One cup of either green or brown lentils, washed and drained, is needed.
- 2 medium sweet potatoes, peeled and diced
- 1 tablespoon garlic-infused oil
- 1 teaspoon ground cumin
- 1 teaspoon ground coriander
- 1/2 teaspoon turmeric
- 1/2 teaspoon ground ginger
- 1/4 teaspoon cayenne pepper (adjust to taste)
- 1 can (14 oz) diced tomatoes
- 1 can (14 oz) coconut milk (use lactose-free if needed)
- 2 cups low-sodium vegetable broth
- 2 cups baby spinach
- Salt and pepper to taste
- Fresh cilantro leaves for garnish

PROCEDURE:

1. **Cooking Lentils and Sweet Potatoes:**
   - In a big pot, warm the garlic-flavored oil over medium heat.
   - Add the diced sweet potatoes and cook for about 5 minutes, stirring occasionally, until they start to soften.
   - Add the ground cumin, ground coriander, turmeric, ground ginger, and cayenne pepper. Stir to coat the sweet potatoes with the spices.
   - Add the rinsed lentils, diced tomatoes (with their juices), coconut milk, and vegetable broth. Stir well to combine.

- Bring the mixture to a boil, then reduce the heat to low, cover the pot, and let it simmer for about 20-25 minutes, or until the lentils and sweet potatoes are tender.

2. **Finishing the Curry:**
   - Once the lentils and sweet potatoes are cooked, stir in the baby spinach and let it wilt into the curry.
   - Add salt and pepper to the curry to your liking.
   - If the curry is too thick, you can add a bit more vegetable broth or water to achieve the desired consistency.

3. **Serving:**
   - Ladle the Lentil and Sweet Potato Curry into serving bowls.
   - For an extra burst of flavor and a pop of color, top off your dish with some fresh cilantro leaves.

NUTRITIONAL VALUE (PER SERVING):

- Calories: 320 kcal
- Carbohydrates: 45g
- Protein: 12g
- Fat: 10g
- Fiber: 10g

HEALTH BENEFITS:

- Low FODMAP: This curry is carefully crafted to follow low FODMAP guidelines, reducing potential triggers for IBS symptoms.
- Lentils: Rich in soluble fiber and plant-based protein, lentils support digestive health and help maintain stable blood sugar levels.
- Sweet Potatoes: These root vegetables are a great source of vitamin A, fiber, and potassium, aiding digestion and promoting gut health.
- Spices: Turmeric, cumin, coriander, and ginger have anti-inflammatory properties that may alleviate IBS-related discomfort.
- Spinach: Baby spinach adds vitamins, minerals, and additional fiber to the dish.

STUFFED BELL PEPPERS WITH QUINOA AND SPINACH

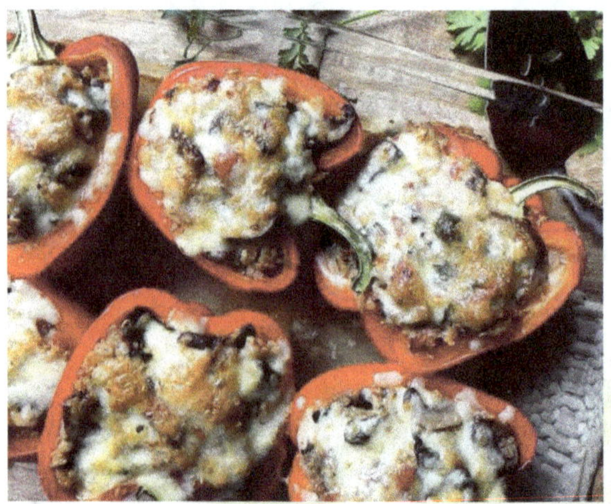

INGREDIENTS:

- 4 large bell peppers, any color
- 1 cup quinoa, rinsed
- 2 cups low-sodium vegetable broth
- 2 cups fresh baby spinach, chopped
- 1 tablespoon garlic-infused oil
- 1 small zucchini, diced
- 1 small carrot, diced
- 1/2 cup crumbled feta cheese (optional; omit for a dairy-free version)
- 1 teaspoon dried oregano
- 1 teaspoon ground cumin
- Salt and pepper to taste
- Olive oil for drizzling
- Fresh parsley leaves for garnish

PROCEDURE:

1. **Prepping the Bell Peppers:**
   - Preheat the oven to 375°F (190°C).
   - Trim the tops of the bell peppers and take out the seeds and inner parts.
   - Put the bell peppers in a baking dish, sprinkle with a little olive oil, and bake in the preheated oven for around 15-20 minutes to make them tender.
2. **Cooking the Quinoa and Filling:**
   - In a saucepan, combine the rinsed quinoa and vegetable broth. Bring to a boil, then reduce the heat to low, cover, and simmer for about 15 minutes, or until the quinoa is cooked and the liquid is absorbed.

- In a skillet, heat the garlic-infused oil over medium heat. Add the diced zucchini and carrot, and sauté for about 5 minutes, until they start to soften.
- Mix in the diced baby spinach and cook until it is limp.
- Add the cooked quinoa, dried oregano, ground cumin, crumbled feta cheese (if using), salt, and pepper. Mix well to combine.

3. **Stuffing the Bell Peppers:**
   - Carefully fill each roasted bell pepper with the quinoa and spinach mixture.
   - Place the stuffed peppers back into the baking dish.
   - Drizzle a touch of olive oil over the stuffed peppers.

4. **Baking and Serving:**
   - Bake the stuffed peppers in the preheated oven for an additional 20-25 minutes, or until the peppers are tender and the filling is heated through.
   - Garnish with fresh parsley leaves before serving.

NUTRITIONAL VALUE (PER SERVING):

- Calories: 280 kcal
- Carbohydrates: 42g
- Protein: 10g
- Fat: 8g
- Fiber: 7g

HEALTH BENEFITS:

- Low FODMAP: These stuffed bell peppers adhere to the low FODMAP principles, minimizing potential triggers for IBS symptoms.
- Quinoa: Rich in fiber and protein, quinoa provides sustained energy and supports digestive regularity.
- Spinach: Baby spinach contributes vitamins, minerals, and fiber that assist in maintaining gut health.
- Bell Peppers: These vibrant vegetables offer vitamin C and antioxidants, potentially aiding inflammation reduction.
- Olive Oil: Drizzling olive oil adds healthy fats that may help soothe the digestive tract.

4

MAIN DISHES: NON-VEGETARIAN

BAKED SALMON WITH ROASTED ASPARAGUS

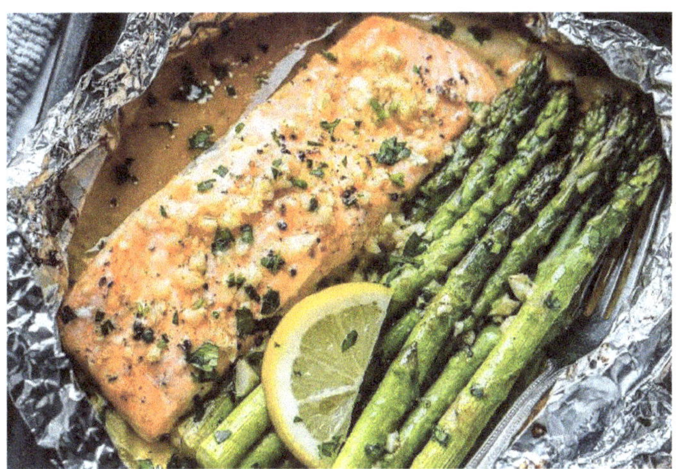

INGREDIENTS:

- 4 salmon fillets (6 oz each), skinless
- 1 bunch of asparagus, trimmed
- 2 tablespoons olive oil
- 1 lemon, thinly sliced
- 2 cloves garlic, minced
- 1 teaspoon fresh dill, chopped
- Salt and pepper to taste

PROCEDURE:

1. **Preparation:**
   - Preheat the oven to 400°F (200°C).
   - Place the salmon fillets on a plate and pat them dry with paper towels. Sprinkle a pinch of salt and pepper over each fillet.

2. **Asparagus Prep:**
   - Arrange the trimmed asparagus on a baking sheet.
   - Coat the ingredients with 1 tablespoon of olive oil, then sprinkle with salt and pepper. Give everything a good mix to make sure it's evenly distributed.

3. **Salmon and Asparagus Bake:**
   - On the same baking sheet, make a little space for the salmon fillets. Place the seasoned salmon fillets on the sheet.
   - Scatter minced garlic and chopped dill over the salmon fillets.
   - Put some lemon slices on top of the salmon.
   - Drizzle the remaining olive oil over the entire sheet.

- Cover the sheet with aluminum foil and bake in the preheated oven for about 15-20 minutes, or until the salmon flakes easily with a fork.

4. **Serve:**
   - Gently remove the aluminum foil and transfer the salmon and asparagus to serving plates.
   - Squeeze a little lemon juice over the salmon before serving.

NUTRITIONAL VALUE (PER SERVING):

- Calories: ~300 kcal
- Protein: ~30g
- Carbohydrates: ~7g
- Dietary Fiber: ~3g
- Total Fat: ~18g
- Saturated Fat: ~3g
- Omega-3 Fatty Acids: ~1,000mg
- Vitamin C: ~30mg
- Vitamin D: ~450IU
- Calcium: ~50mg

HEALTH BENEFITS:

- Salmon is rich in omega-3 fatty acids, which have anti-inflammatory properties that may help soothe IBS symptoms.
- Asparagus is a low-FODMAP vegetable, making it gentle on the digestive system and less likely to trigger IBS symptoms.
- Garlic is used in moderation to add flavor; it's a potential prebiotic that could support a balanced gut microbiome.
- Lemon provides a burst of vitamin C, which supports immune health and aids digestion.
- Olive oil offers heart-healthy monounsaturated fats that are well-tolerated by most IBS sufferers.
- Dill not only enhances flavor but also has anti-inflammatory properties.

GRILLED TURKEY BURGERS WITH AVOCADO SALSA

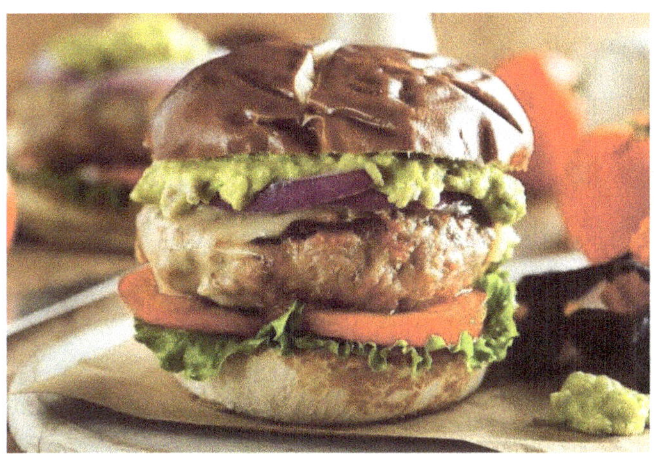

INGREDIENTS:

- **For the Turkey Burgers:**
- 1 pound ground turkey
- 1/4 cup gluten-free breadcrumbs
- 1 teaspoon garlic powder
- 1 teaspoon ground cumin
- 1/2 teaspoon paprika
- Salt and pepper to taste
- **For the Avocado Salsa:**
- 2 ripe avocados, diced
- 1/2 cup diced tomato
- 1/4 cup chopped fresh cilantro
- 1/4 cup finely chopped red onion
- 1 small jalapeno, seeds removed and finely chopped
- Juice of 1 lime
- Salt to taste

PROCEDURE:

1. **Turkey Burger Prep:**
   - In a bowl, combine ground turkey, gluten-free breadcrumbs, garlic powder, ground cumin, paprika, salt, and pepper.
   - Gently stir the ingredients together until everything is blended, taking care not to overmix the meat.
2. **Forming Patties:**
   - Divide the turkey mixture into 4 equal portions.

- Shape each portion into a burger patty, ensuring they are evenly sized for even cooking.

3. **Grilling the Patties:**
   - Preheat the grill to medium-high heat.
   - Place the turkey patties on the grill and cook for about 5-6 minutes per side, or until the internal temperature reaches 165°F (75°C) and the burgers are no longer pink in the center.

4. **Avocado Salsa Prep:**
   - In a bowl, combine the diced avocados, diced tomato, chopped cilantro, finely chopped red onion, and jalapeno.
   - Pour the lime juice over the mixture and give it a gentle stir to mix everything together.
   - Season the salsa with a pinch of salt, adjusting to taste.

5. **Assembling the Burgers:**
   - Place the grilled turkey burgers on gluten-free buns or lettuce wraps.
   - Top each burger with a generous portion of avocado salsa.

NUTRITIONAL VALUE (PER SERVING):

- Calories: ~300 kcal
- Protein: ~25g
- Carbohydrates: ~15g
- Dietary Fiber: ~7g
- Total Fat: ~18g
- Saturated Fat: ~3g
- Vitamin A: ~1000IU
- Vitamin C: ~20mg
- Folate: ~40mcg
- Potassium: ~600mg

HEALTH BENEFITS:

- Ground turkey is a lean protein source that's easier to digest compared to fatty meats, making it suitable for IBS patients.
- Gluten-free breadcrumbs are gentle on the digestive system, minimizing potential triggers.
- Spices like garlic powder, cumin, and paprika add flavor without excess heat, suitable for sensitive stomachs.
- Avocado is a low-FODMAP fruit rich in healthy fats, which can provide sustained energy and support digestive health.

- Tomatoes and onions, when consumed in moderation, offer vitamins and antioxidants without overloading the gut.
- Cilantro and lime provide refreshing flavors without causing discomfort.

LEMON-GARLIC SHRIMP STIR-FRY

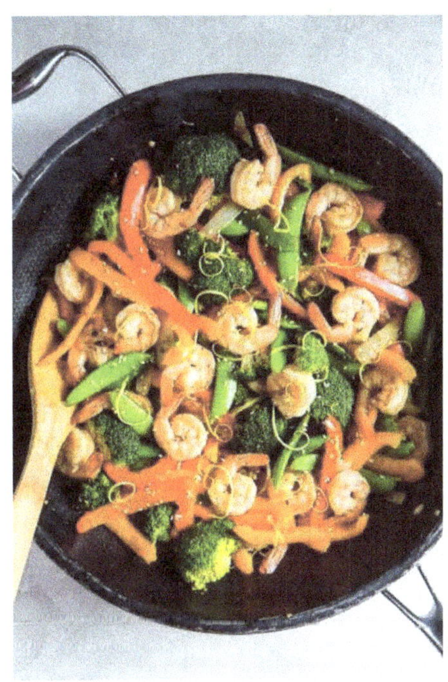

INGREDIENTS:

- **For the Stir-Fry:**
- 1 pound medium shrimp, peeled and deveined
- 2 cups mixed bell peppers, sliced
- 1 cup zucchini, sliced
- 1 cup carrots, julienned
- 1 cup green beans, trimmed and halved
- 2 tablespoons olive oil
- Salt and pepper to taste
- **For the Lemon-Garlic Sauce:**
- Juice of 2 lemons
- 3 cloves garlic, minced

- 2 tablespoons low-sodium chicken broth
- 1 teaspoon grated lemon zest
- 1 tablespoon fresh parsley, chopped

PROCEDURE:

1. **Preparation:**
   - In a bowl, combine the shrimp with a pinch of salt, pepper, and minced garlic. Allow the flavors to marinate for about 10 minutes.
2. **Stir-Fry:**
   - In a big skillet or wok, warm up 1 tablespoon of olive oil over medium-high heat.
   - Add the mixed bell peppers, zucchini, carrots, and green beans to the skillet. Stir-fry for about 4-5 minutes, or until the vegetables are slightly tender.
   - Take them out of the skillet and put them aside.
3. **Cooking the Shrimp:**
   - In the same skillet, add the remaining tablespoon of olive oil. Once hot, add the marinated shrimp.
   - Cook the shrimp for about 2-3 minutes on each side, or until they turn pink and opaque.
4. **Preparing the Sauce:**
   - In a small bowl, whisk together the lemon juice, low-sodium chicken broth, and grated lemon zest.
   - Pour the lemon-garlic sauce over the cooked shrimp in the skillet.
5. **Combining and Serving:**
   - Put the cooked vegetables back in the skillet with the shrimp.
   - Gently toss the ingredients to coat them with the lemon-garlic sauce.
   - Sprinkle fresh chopped parsley over the stir-fry before serving.

NUTRITIONAL VALUE (PER SERVING):

- Calories: ~250 kcal
- Protein: ~20g
- Carbohydrates: ~15g
- Dietary Fiber: ~5g
- Total Fat: ~12g
- Saturated Fat: ~2g
- Vitamin C: ~70mg
- Vitamin A: ~1500IU
- Vitamin K: ~50mcg
- Folate: ~50mcg

- Potassium: ~500mg

HEALTH BENEFITS:

- Shrimp is a lean protein source with minimal fat content, making it suitable for IBS patients.
- Mixed bell peppers, zucchini, carrots, and green beans are low-FODMAP vegetables, providing essential nutrients without triggering IBS symptoms.
- Olive oil is a healthy fat that can be well-tolerated by most IBS individuals, contributing to satiety and overall wellness.
- Lemon juice and zest add a burst of flavor without causing digestive distress.
- Garlic is used in moderation, providing flavor and potential prebiotic benefits.
- Fresh parsley not only enhances taste but also offers a touch of digestive comfort.

5

SIDES AND SNACK

ROASTED TURMERIC CAULIFLOWER BITES

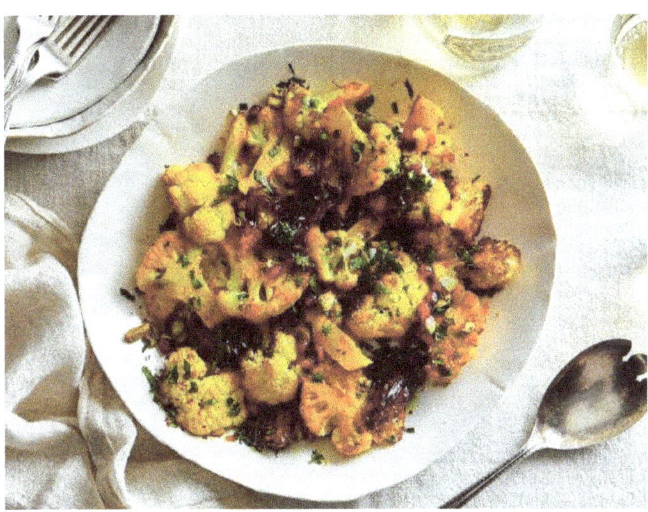

INGREDIENTS:

- One medium-sized head of cauliflower, cut into small pieces.
- 2 tablespoons olive oil
- 1 teaspoon ground turmeric
- 1/2 teaspoon ground cumin
- 1/2 teaspoon paprika
- 1/4 teaspoon cayenne pepper (adjust to taste)
- Salt and pepper to taste
- Fresh parsley, chopped, for garnish

PROCEDURE:

- Preheat your oven to 400°F (200°C).
- In a large mixing bowl, combine the olive oil, ground turmeric, ground cumin, paprika, cayenne pepper, salt, and pepper. Mix well to create a marinade.
- Add the cauliflower florets to the bowl and toss them until evenly coated with the marinade.
- Spread the cauliflower florets in a single layer on a baking sheet lined with parchment paper.

- Ensure that the items are not too close together so that they can be cooked evenly.
- Roast the cauliflower in the preheated oven for 20-25 minutes or until they are tender and golden brown, tossing them halfway through to ensure even cooking.

- Once the cauliflower has been roasted to perfection, take it out of the oven and let it cool off a bit.
- Garnish the roasted cauliflower bites with freshly chopped parsley before serving.

NUTRITIONAL VALUE (PER SERVING):

- Calories: 80
- Total Fat: 6g
- Saturated Fat: 1g
- Cholesterol: 0mg
- Sodium: 150mg
- Total Carbohydrates: 7g
- Dietary Fiber: 3g
- Sugars: 2g
- Protein: 2g

HEALTH BENEFITS:

- Cauliflower: A low-FODMAP (fermentable oligosaccharides, disaccharides, monosaccharides, and polyols) vegetable, cauliflower is gentle on the digestive system for IBS sufferers. It's rich in fiber, vitamins, and minerals while being easily digestible.
- Turmeric: Curcumin, the active compound in turmeric, has anti-inflammatory properties that may help soothe inflammation and discomfort associated with IBS. It can also aid digestion and support overall gut health.
- Cumin: Cumin is known to have carminative properties, which means it can help alleviate gas and bloating.It gives the dish a delightful taste.
- Paprika: Paprika adds a burst of flavor without causing digestive distress. It's a source of antioxidants and may have anti-inflammatory effects.
- Olive Oil: A source of heart-healthy monounsaturated fats, olive oil is well-tolerated by many IBS individuals. It helps in absorbing fat-soluble vitamins and supports a healthy gut lining.
- Cayenne Pepper: The capsaicin in cayenne pepper can stimulate digestion and promote bowel regularity. However, its spiciness might trigger symptoms in some people, so adjust the amount according to your tolerance.

CUCUMBER AND CARROT STICKS WITH HUMMUS

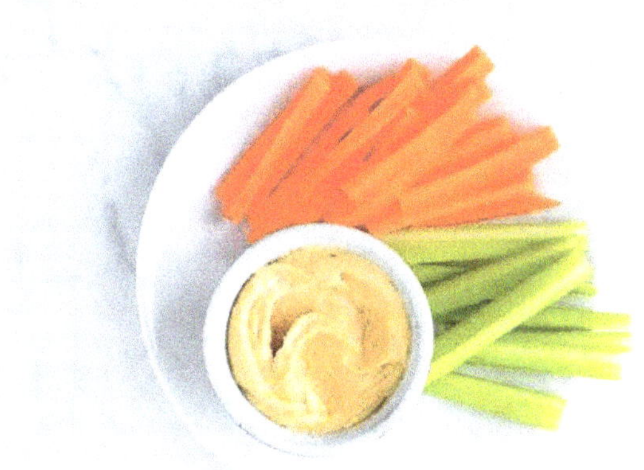

INGREDIENTS:

- 2 medium cucumbers, washed and cut into sticks
- 2 large carrots, peeled and cut into sticks
- **For Hummus:**
- One 15-ounce can of chickpeas, drained and rinsed.
- 3 tablespoons tahini
- 3 tablespoons lemon juice
- 2 cloves garlic, minced
- 1/2 teaspoon ground cumin
- 1/4 teaspoon paprika
- 2 tablespoons olive oil
- Salt and pepper to taste
- Water (as needed to achieve desired consistency)
- Fresh parsley, chopped, for garnish

PROCEDURE:

- In a food processor, combine the chickpeas, tahini, lemon juice, minced garlic, ground cumin, paprika, olive oil, salt, and pepper.
- Blend the mixture until smooth, adding water gradually to reach your preferred hummus consistency. Adjust the seasonings as needed.
- Transfer the hummus to a serving bowl, drizzle with a little olive oil, and sprinkle with paprika and chopped parsley for garnish.
- Arrange the cucumber and carrot sticks on a platter alongside the bowl of hummus.

NUTRITIONAL VALUE (PER SERVING, INCLUDING HUMMUS):

- Calories: 180
- Total Fat: 9g
- Saturated Fat: 1g
- Cholesterol: 0mg
- Sodium: 200mg
- Total Carbohydrates: 22g
- Dietary Fiber: 7g
- Sugars: 4g
- Protein: 7g

HEALTH BENEFITS

- Cucumber: Cucumbers are hydrating and low in FODMAPs, making them suitable for IBS. Their high water content can help maintain hydration and support regular bowel movements.
- Carrots: Carrots are a good source of soluble fiber, which can promote digestive regularity and soothe IBS symptoms. They are generally well-tolerated and provide essential vitamins and antioxidants.
- Chickpeas: Chickpeas are rich in soluble fiber and protein. When well-cooked and consumed in moderation, they can be a part of a low-FODMAP diet, aiding in gut health and satiety.
- Tahini: Made from sesame seeds, tahini is a good source of healthy fats and provides a creamy texture to the hummus. It adds flavor and nutrients, including calcium and iron.
- Lemon Juice: Lemon juice's acidity can stimulate digestive juices, aiding in digestion. It also provides a burst of vitamin C, an antioxidant that supports the immune system.
- Garlic (small amount): While garlic can be a trigger for some IBS sufferers, using a small amount of minced garlic in the hummus might be tolerable, as its strong flavor is diluted.
- Olive Oil: Incorporating olive oil in moderation can provide monounsaturated fats that support heart health and potentially reduce inflammation in the gut.
- Cumin: Cumin's carminative properties may help alleviate gas and bloating, enhancing overall comfort during digestion.

HERBED QUINOA SALAD

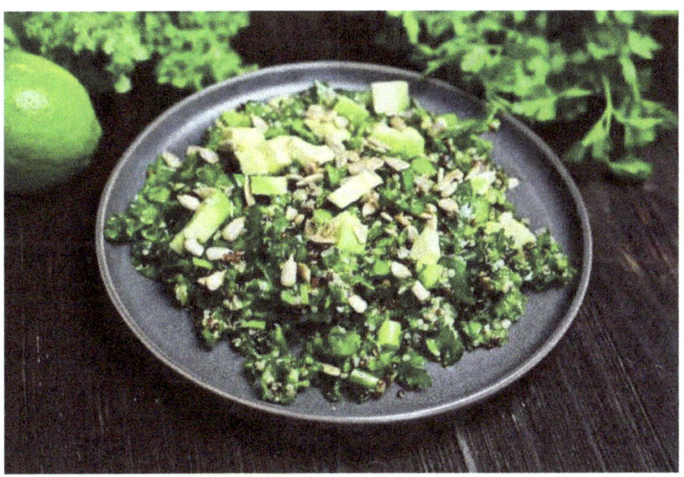

INGREDIENTS:

- 1 cup quinoa, rinsed and drained
- 2 cups water or low-sodium vegetable broth
- 1 cup cherry tomatoes, halved
- 1 cucumber, diced
- 1 red bell pepper, diced
- 1/4 red onion, finely chopped
- 1/4 cup fresh parsley, chopped
- 2 tablespoons fresh mint, chopped
- 1/4 cup feta cheese, crumbled (optional)
- **For the Dressing:**
- 3 tablespoons extra-virgin olive oil
- 2 tablespoons lemon juice
- 1 teaspoon Dijon mustard
- Salt and pepper to taste

PROCEDURE:

- In a medium-sized saucepan, bring the water or vegetable broth to a boil. Once boiling, add the quinoa and reduce the heat to low. Cover the pan and let it simmer for around 15 minutes, or until the quinoa is cooked and the liquid is absorbed.
- Take the saucepan off the heat and let the quinoa sit, covered, for a period of five minutes. Fluff the quinoa with a fork and let it cool to room temperature.
- In a large mixing bowl, combine the cooked quinoa, cherry tomatoes, cucumber, red bell pepper, red onion, parsley, mint, and feta cheese (if using).

- In a small bowl, whisk together the extra-virgin olive oil, lemon juice, Dijon mustard, salt, and pepper to create the dressing.
- Drizzle the dressing over the quinoa and vegetable mixture. Toss well to combine, ensuring all ingredients are coated with the dressing.
- Taste and adjust the seasoning if needed. You can refrigerate the salad for about 30 minutes before serving to allow the flavors to meld.
- Serve the herbed quinoa salad cold, garnished with additional fresh herbs if desired.

NUTRITIONAL VALUE (PER SERVING):

- Calories: 220
- Total Fat: 10g
- Saturated Fat: 2g
- Cholesterol: 5mg
- Sodium: 190mg
- Total Carbohydrates: 28g
- Dietary Fiber: 4g
- Sugars: 3g
- Protein: 6g

HEALTH BENEFITS

- Quinoa: Quinoa is a gluten-free whole grain that's gentle on the digestive system. It's a great source of fiber and protein, offering sustained energy without causing digestive discomfort.
- Cherry Tomatoes: Cherry tomatoes are low in FODMAPs and provide vitamins A and C, as well as antioxidants that can support a healthy gut.
- Cucumber: Cucumbers have a high water content that helps with hydration, while their low FODMAP content makes them suitable for IBS. They're also easy to digest.
- Red Bell Pepper: Low in FODMAPs and high in vitamins, red bell peppers add color and crunch to the salad. They contain antioxidants that promote gut health.
- Red Onion (small amount): In moderation, red onion can be tolerated by some individuals with IBS. It adds flavor and a mild prebiotic effect that supports gut bacteria.
- Fresh Herbs (Parsley and Mint): Herbs are typically well-tolerated and add a burst of flavor to the dish. Parsley and mint can aid digestion and add a refreshing touch.
- Extra-Virgin Olive Oil: The healthy fats in olive oil can contribute to a well-balanced diet. They may help reduce inflammation and support gut lining integrity.
- Lemon Juice: Lemon juice's acidity aids digestion and can enhance the flavor of the salad.
- It's also a great source of vitamin C and antioxidants.

6

BREADS AND WRAP

GLUTEN-FREE OAT BREAD

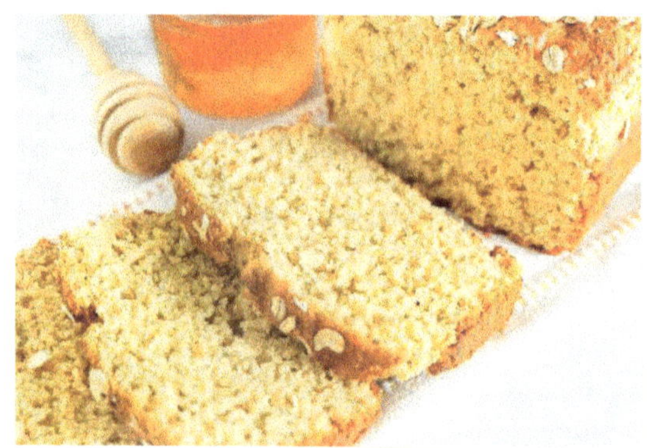

INGREDIENTS:

- 2 cups gluten-free oat flour
- 1 cup almond flour
- 1/2 cup ground flaxseed
- 1/4 cup chia seeds
- 1 teaspoon baking soda
- 1/2 teaspoon salt
- 4 large eggs
- 1/4 cup olive oil
- 1 tablespoon apple cider vinegar
- 1 cup unsweetened almond milk
- 2 tablespoons honey (optional)
- 1/2 cup chopped walnuts (optional)

PROCEDURE:

- Preheat your oven to 350°F (175°C) and grease a 9x5-inch loaf pan.
- In a large mixing bowl, combine the gluten-free oat flour, almond flour, ground flaxseed, chia seeds, baking soda, and salt.
- In a separate bowl, whisk together the eggs, olive oil, apple cider vinegar, almond milk, and honey (if using).
- Gradually incorporate the wet ingredients into the dry ingredients, stirring until a consistent batter is created. If you'd like, you can mix in the chopped walnuts.
- Pour the mixture into the prepped loaf pan and make sure it is spread out evenly.
- Bake in the preheated oven for 45-50 minutes or until a toothpick inserted into the center of the bread comes out clean.
- Once the bread is done baking, take it out of the oven and let it sit in the pan for around 10 minutes. After that, move it to a wire rack to cool off completely before cutting it.

NUTRITIONAL VALUE (PER SERVING):

- (Based on 1 slice, assuming 12 slices per loaf)
- Calories: ~180 kcal
- Total Fat: 12g
- Saturated Fat: 1.5g
- Cholesterol: 70mg
- Sodium: 210mg
- Total Carbohydrates: 12g
- Dietary Fiber: 4g
- Sugars: 2g
- Protein: 6g

HEALTH BENEFITS:

- Gluten-Free: This oat bread is free from gluten, making it suitable for individuals with gluten sensitivity or celiac disease, common among those with IBS.
- Rich in Fiber: Oats, flaxseed, and chia seeds are excellent sources of dietary fiber. Fiber promotes healthy digestion, helps prevent constipation, and can contribute to managing IBS symptoms.
- Healthy Fats: Almond flour and olive oil provide heart-healthy monounsaturated fats, supporting overall heart health and reducing inflammation.
- Protein Content: With a moderate protein content, this bread can aid in maintaining muscle mass and providing a steady source of energy.
- Omega-3 Fatty Acids: Flaxseed and chia seeds are rich in omega-3 fatty acids, which have anti-inflammatory properties and could potentially alleviate some IBS symptoms.
- Low Sugar: The minimal sugar content ensures stable blood sugar levels, important for individuals with IBS to avoid triggering digestive issues.
- Nutrient Density: This bread contains vitamins, minerals, and antioxidants from the various ingredients, contributing to overall health and wellness.

BROWN RICE TORTILLAS

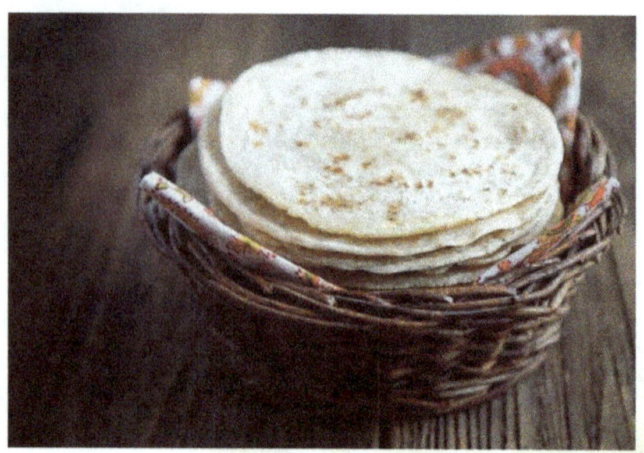

INGREDIENTS:

- 1 cup brown rice flour
- 1/4 cup tapioca flour
- 1/2 teaspoon salt
- 1/2 teaspoon baking powder
- 2 tablespoons olive oil
- 1/2 cup warm water

PROCEDURE:

- In a mixing bowl, combine the brown rice flour, tapioca flour, salt, and baking powder.
- Pour the olive oil into the dry ingredients and stir until the combination is crumbly.
- Gradually add warm water while stirring.
- Knead the mixture until it becomes a soft, pliable dough. If the dough is too dry, add a bit more water; if too wet, add a touch of brown rice flour.
- Divide the dough into small balls, about golf ball size.
- Roll out each ball between two sheets of parchment paper to your desired tortilla thickness.
- Heat a non-stick skillet over medium heat.
- Carefully peel off the top parchment paper from a rolled-out dough circle and place the tortilla, parchment side up, onto the heated skillet.
- Once the tortilla begins to bubble and the edges lift slightly (after about 1-2 minutes), carefully peel off the parchment paper.
- Cook the tortilla for another 1-2 minutes until the underside is lightly browned and slightly crispy, then flip it and cook the other side.
- Remove the tortilla from the skillet and place it between a clean kitchen towel to keep it soft and pliable. Do the same thing with the other dough balls.

NUTRITIONAL VALUE (PER TORTILLA):

- (Recipe makes approximately 6 tortillas)
- Calories: ~140 kcal
- Total Fat: 5g
- Saturated Fat: 0.5g
- Cholesterol: 0mg
- Sodium: 200mg
- Total Carbohydrates: 22g
- Dietary Fiber: 1g
- Sugars: 0g
- Protein: 1g

HEALTH BENEFITS:

- Gluten-Free: Brown rice flour and tapioca flour are naturally gluten-free, making these tortillas suitable for those with gluten sensitivity or celiac disease, common among individuals with IBS.
- Gentle on the Gut: Brown rice is a complex carbohydrate that is generally well-tolerated by individuals with IBS, as it's less likely to cause digestive distress compared to refined grains.
- Low-FODMAP: Brown rice is considered a low-FODMAP food, which means it's less likely to trigger IBS symptoms in sensitive individuals.
- Digestive-Friendly: The combination of brown rice and tapioca flour can provide a smoother digestion experience, reducing the risk of bloating and discomfort.
- Minimal Additives: Making your own tortillas allows you to control the ingredients, avoiding additives and preservatives that might aggravate IBS symptoms.
- Nutrient Content: While these tortillas are not high in protein, they still provide essential carbohydrates and a small amount of healthy fats.
- Versatile: These tortillas can be used for wraps, tacos, quesadillas, and other dishes, providing a flexible base for a variety of fillings.

SPINACH AND FETA STUFFED FLATBREAD

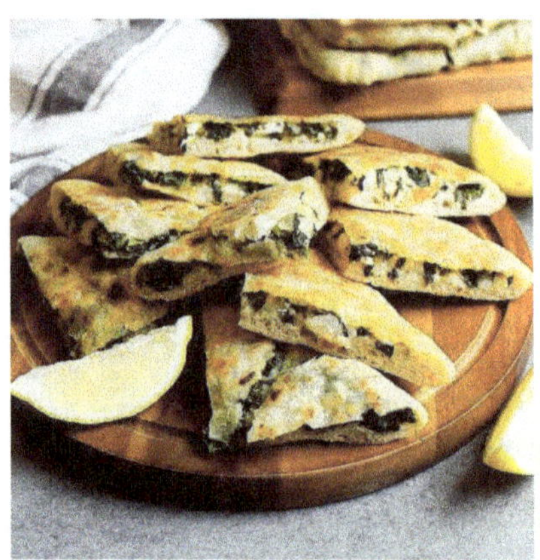

INGREDIENTS:

- **For the Flatbread:**
- 2 cups gluten-free all-purpose flour
- 1 teaspoon baking powder
- 1/2 teaspoon salt
- 1/4 cup olive oil
- 3/4 cup warm water
- **For the Filling:**
- 2 cups fresh spinach, chopped
- 1/2 cup crumbled feta cheese
- 1/4 cup chopped green onions (green parts only)
- 1/4 teaspoon black pepper
- 1/4 teaspoon garlic powder

PROCEDURE:

1. **For the Flatbread:**
   - In a large mixing bowl, whisk together the gluten-free all-purpose flour, baking powder, and salt.
   - Combine the olive oil and warm water with the dry ingredients, stirring until a dough is formed.
   - Knead the dough for a few minutes until it is soft and stretchy.
   - Divide the dough into equal-sized balls (about 6-8 balls) and cover them with a damp cloth.
   - Allow them to take a break for approximately 15-20 minutes.
   - Roll out each ball into a thin round flatbread using a rolling pin.
2. **For the Filling:**

- In a mixing bowl, combine the chopped spinach, crumbled feta cheese, chopped green onions, black pepper, and garlic powder. Mix well.

3. **Assembly:**
   - Place a portion of the filling onto one half of each rolled-out flatbread.
   - Fold the remaining flatbread over the filling to form a semi-circle.Press down the edges to seal the flatbread.
   - Warm up a non-stick skillet or griddle on medium heat.
   - Place the stuffed flatbread onto the skillet and cook for about 2-3 minutes on each side, or until the flatbread is golden brown and the filling is heated through.
   - Take the skillet off the heat and let it cool down a bit before serving.

NUTRITIONAL VALUE (PER STUFFED FLATBREAD):

- (Recipe makes approximately 6 stuffed flatbreads)
- Calories: ~240 kcal
- Total Fat: 10g
- Saturated Fat: 3.5g
- Cholesterol: 15mg
- Sodium: 390mg
- Total Carbohydrates: 30g
- Dietary Fiber: 3g
- Sugars: 1g
- Protein: 7g

HEALTH BENEFITS:

- Gluten-Free Option: The gluten-free all-purpose flour used in the flatbread ensures that individuals with gluten sensitivity or celiac disease can enjoy this dish without triggering symptoms.
- IBS-Friendly Ingredients: Fresh spinach, green onions (green parts), and feta cheese are generally considered low-FODMAP ingredients, making them suitable for those following an IBS elimination diet.
- Leafy Greens: Spinach is rich in vitamins, minerals, and antioxidants, which can support overall gut health and reduce inflammation often associated with IBS.
- Protein and Healthy Fat: Feta cheese provides a source of protein and healthy fats, contributing to satiety and balanced energy levels.
- Digestive Benefits: This dish includes ingredients that are less likely to cause digestive discomfort, such as garlic powder rather than fresh garlic.
- Flavorful and Satisfying: The combination of spinach and feta creates a flavorful and satisfying filling for the flatbread, making it a tasty option for a light meal or snack.

7

DRESSINGS AND SAUCES

CREAMY AVOCADO DRESSING

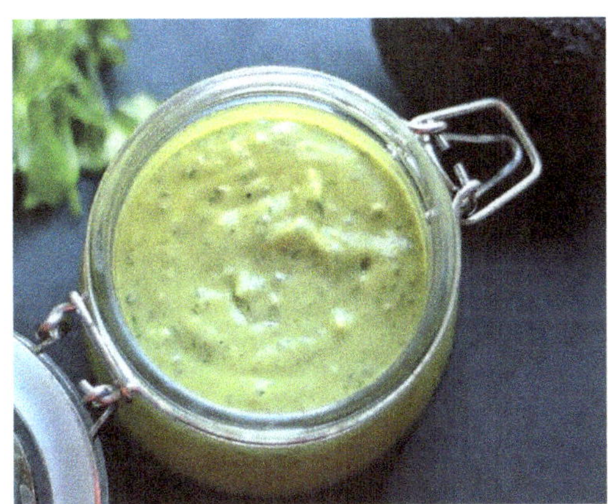

INGREDIENTS:

- 1 ripe avocado, peeled and pitted
- 1/4 cup plain lactose-free yogurt
- 2 tablespoons fresh lemon juice
- 2 tablespoons extra-virgin olive oil
- 1 small garlic clove, minced
- 1/4 teaspoon ground cumin
- Salt and pepper to taste
- 2-4 tablespoons water (adjust for desired consistency)

PROCEDURE:

- In a blender or food processor, combine the avocado, lactose-free yogurt, lemon juice, olive oil, minced garlic, ground cumin, salt, and pepper.
- Blend the ingredients on medium speed until a smooth and creamy consistency is achieved.
- If the dressing seems too thick, gradually add water while blending until the desired thickness is reached.
- Taste and adjust seasoning as needed, adding more salt, pepper, or lemon juice according to your preference.
- Move the dressing to a container and keep it in the fridge until you're ready to use it. The dressing can be kept for up to 3 days.

NUTRITIONAL VALUE (PER SERVING):

- Calories: approximately 100 kcal
- Total Fat: 9g
- Saturated Fat: 1g

- Carbohydrates: 4g
- Fiber: 3g
- Protein: 1g
- Vitamin K: 25% of the Recommended Daily Intake (RDI)
- Folate: 15% of the RDI
- Vitamin C: 10% of the RDI
- Potassium: 8% of the RDI

HEALTH BENEFITS:

- IBS-Friendly: The Creamy Avocado Dressing is gentle on the digestive system due to its use of lactose-free yogurt and easily digestible avocado. It fits well within the IBS elimination diet guidelines.
- Rich in Healthy Fats: Avocado and olive oil provide heart-healthy monounsaturated fats, which can support overall cardiovascular health.
- Fiber Content: Avocado contributes soluble fiber that supports gut health and may help manage IBS symptoms such as bloating and irregular bowel movements.
- Vitamins and Minerals: The dressing is a source of vitamin K, which plays a role in blood clotting, and folate, which is essential for cell division and repair.
- Anti-Inflammatory: Avocado and olive oil contain compounds with potential anti-inflammatory effects, which can be beneficial for individuals with IBS.
- Creaminess without Dairy: Lactose-free yogurt offers creaminess without triggering lactose intolerance symptoms, making it a suitable option for those with IBS and dairy sensitivities.

GUT-SOOTHING GINGER TURMERIC SAUCE

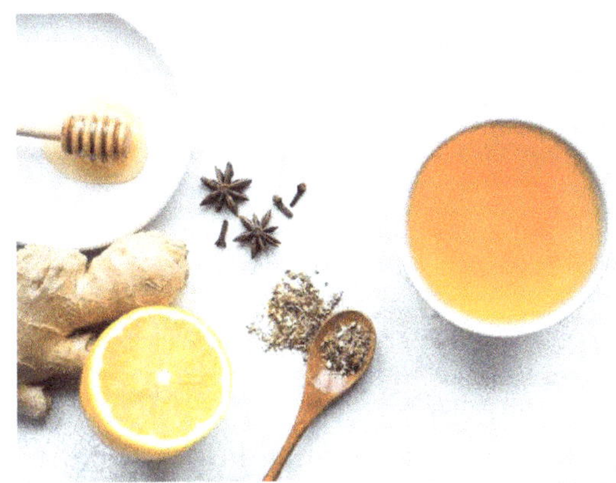

INGREDIENTS:

- 1-inch fresh ginger root, peeled and minced
- 1 teaspoon ground turmeric
- 2 tablespoons extra-virgin olive oil
- 1 tablespoon maple syrup (or honey, if preferred)
- 1 teaspoon apple cider vinegar
- 1/2 teaspoon ground cumin
- 1/4 teaspoon ground black pepper
- Pinch of sea salt
- 2-4 tablespoons water (adjust for desired consistency)

PROCEDURE:

- In a small saucepan, heat the extra-virgin olive oil over low heat.
- Add the minced ginger and sauté for a couple of minutes until fragrant.
- Stir in the ground turmeric, ground cumin, ground black pepper, and a pinch of sea salt.

- Stir for an additional minute to blend the flavors.
- Take the saucepan off the heat and let the mixture cool down a bit.
- Pour the mixture into a blender or food processor.Add the maple syrup, apple cider vinegar, and a couple of tablespoons of water.
- Blend the mixture on medium speed until a smooth and vibrant sauce is achieved.
- If necessary, add more liquid to get the desired consistency.
- Taste and adjust the seasoning, adding more salt or maple syrup as per your preference.
- Once blended to your satisfaction, transfer the sauce to a glass container.
- It can be kept in the fridge for up to seven days.

NUTRITIONAL VALUE (PER SERVING):

- Calories: approximately 50 kcal
- Total Fat: 4g
- Saturated Fat: 0.5g
- Carbohydrates: 4g
- Fiber: 0.5g
- Sugars: 2g
- Vitamin C: 2% of the Recommended Daily Intake (RDI)
- Iron: 4% of the RDI
- Curcumin (from turmeric): Contains bioactive compounds with potential health benefits, including anti-inflammatory properties.

HEALTH BENEFITS:

- Anti-Inflammatory Magic: The combination of ginger and turmeric brings a potent anti-inflammatory punch, which can help soothe inflammation in the digestive tract, offering relief to those with IBS.
- Gut Comfort: Ginger, known for its anti-nausea properties, may alleviate symptoms like nausea and discomfort often experienced by individuals with IBS.
- Digestive Aid: Ginger has been used traditionally to support digestion and alleviate bloating, making it a helpful ally for IBS symptom management.
- Curcumin's Power: Curcumin, the active compound in turmeric, holds potential to reduce gut inflammation and oxidative stress, contributing to IBS symptom relief.
- Natural Sweetness: The touch of maple syrup adds natural sweetness without overly spiking blood sugar levels, making it suitable for IBS dietary considerations.
- Digestive Tract Support: The inclusion of apple cider vinegar can aid digestion and support a balanced gut environment.

BALSAMIC GLAZE WITH MAPLE AND DIJON

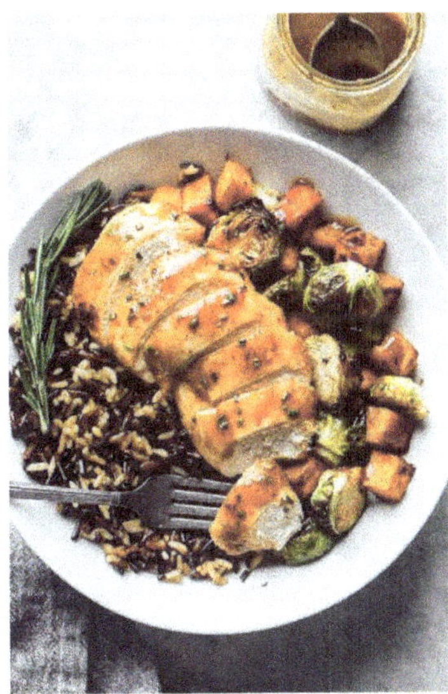

INGREDIENTS:

- 1 cup balsamic vinegar
- 2 tablespoons pure maple syrup
- 1 tablespoon Dijon mustard
- Pinch of sea salt
- Pinch of black pepper

PROCEDURE:

- In a small saucepan, combine the balsamic vinegar and pure maple syrup.
- Put the saucepan on the stove over medium heat and let the mixture come to a gentle boil.
- Reduce the heat to low and let the mixture simmer for about 15-20 minutes, or until it has reduced by about half. The combination should be thick enough to stick to the back of a spoon.
- Remove the saucepan from heat and whisk in the Dijon mustard, sea salt, and black pepper.
- As it cools, the glaze will become thicker.
- Let the glaze cool completely before transferring it to a glass container.
- Store the Balsamic Glaze with Maple and Dijon in the refrigerator. It can be kept for up to two weeks.

NUTRITIONAL VALUE (PER SERVING):

- Calories: approximately 40 kcal
- Total Fat: 0g

- Saturated Fat: 0g
- Carbohydrates: 10g
- Sugars: 9g
- Sodium: 70mg
- Potassium: 2% of the Recommended Daily Intake (RDI)

HEALTH BENEFITS:

Low in Fat: The glaze is naturally low in fat, which aligns well with the IBS elimination diet's focus on gentle and easily digestible foods.

Flavorful Touch: The combination of balsamic vinegar, pure maple syrup, and Dijon mustard provides a harmonious balance of flavors that can elevate the taste of a wide range of dishes.

Gut-Friendly Sweetener: Pure maple syrup, used in moderation, offers a natural sweetness without causing rapid spikes in blood sugar levels, making it suitable for those with IBS.

Digestive Ease: Dijon mustard's slight tanginess can stimulate digestion and potentially aid in alleviating symptoms like bloating and discomfort.

Anti-Inflammatory Potential: Balsamic vinegar contains antioxidants and may have anti-inflammatory effects, contributing to gut health and overall well-being.

Versatility: This glaze is incredibly versatile; it can be used to drizzle over salads, roasted vegetables, grilled meats, and even as a dip for bread.

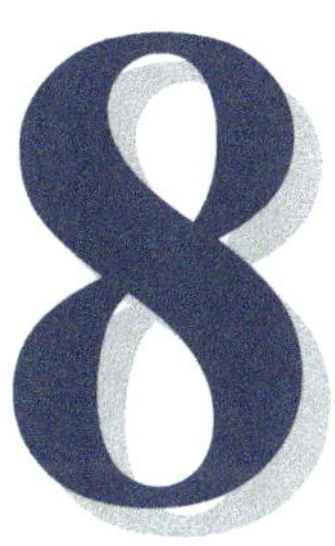

BEVERAGES

MINTY GINGER ICED TEA

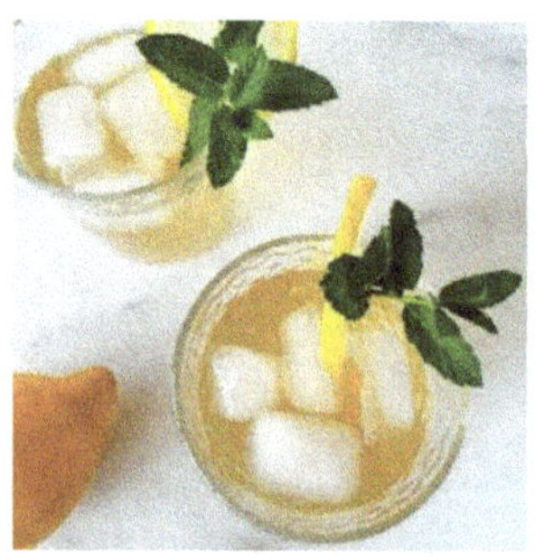

INGREDIENTS:

- 2 cups of water
- 2 green tea bags (caffeine-free)
- 1 tablespoon fresh ginger (peeled and chopped)
- 1 tablespoon fresh mint leaves (chopped)
- 1 teaspoon honey (optional, for sweetness)
- Ice cubes
- For a finishing touch, why not add some fresh mint sprigs and lemon slices?

PROCEDURE:

- Boil 2 cups of water and steep 2 green tea bags in it for about 5 minutes. This ensures a gentle brew that won't aggravate IBS symptoms.
- Remove the tea bags and allow the brewed tea to cool down.
- In a blender, combine the chopped fresh ginger and mint leaves. Add a small amount of the brewed tea to help with blending.
- Blend the ginger and mint mixture until you get a smooth paste.
- Strain the paste through a fine sieve or cheesecloth into a pitcher to remove any solid particles.
- Add the remaining cooled green tea to the pitcher, and stir in 1 teaspoon of honey if desired. Honey can add a touch of sweetness without causing IBS flare-ups.
- Put the mixture in the fridge for at least an hour so that the flavors can combine.
- To serve, fill glasses with ice cubes and pour the minty ginger iced tea over the ice.
- Garnish with fresh mint sprigs and lemon slices for an extra burst of flavor.

NUTRITIONAL VALUE PER SERVING:

- Calories: Approximately 10-15 kcal
- Carbohydrates: 2-3 g
- Fiber: 0.5 g
- Sugars: 1-2 g

- Protein: 0 g
- Fat: 0 g
- Sodium: 5 mg
- Potassium: 30 mg

HEALTH BENEFITS FOR IBS:

- Ginger: Known for its anti-inflammatory and digestive properties, ginger can help soothe gastrointestinal discomfort often experienced by those with IBS.
- Mint: Mint has been traditionally used to relieve symptoms of IBS such as bloating and gas.
- It has a soothing impact on the digestive system.
- Green Tea: Caffeine-free green tea is gentle on the stomach and contains antioxidants that can support overall gut health.
- Honey: While moderation is key, a touch of honey can provide natural sweetness and even have potential anti-inflammatory benefits.
- Hydration: Staying hydrated is crucial for managing IBS. Minty ginger iced tea offers hydration along with soothing properties.

GOLDEN MILK TURMERIC LATTE

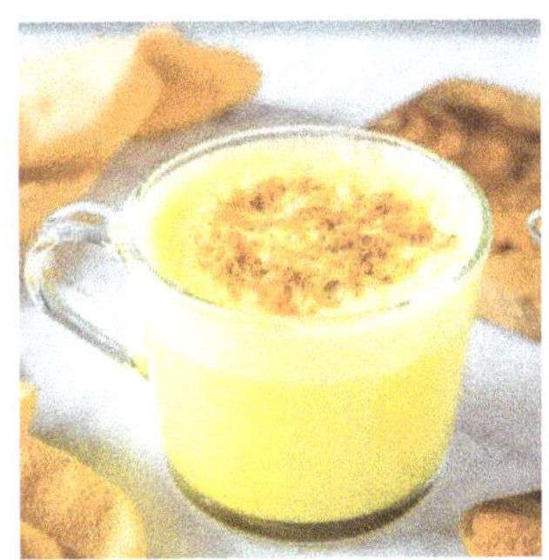

INGREDIENTS:

- 1 cup of unsweetened almond milk (or any preferred non-dairy milk)
- 1 teaspoon ground turmeric
- 1/2 teaspoon ground ginger
- 1/4 teaspoon ground cinnamon
- A pinch of ground black pepper (helps with turmeric absorption)
- 1 teaspoon coconut oil (optional, for creaminess)
- 1 teaspoon honey or maple syrup (optional, for sweetness)
- A dash of ground cardamom (optional, for extra flavor)

- For a bit of spice, you can add a pinch of cayenne pepper (optional).

PROCEDURE:

- In a small saucepan, gently heat the unsweetened almond milk over low to medium heat. Be careful not to boil it.
- Add the ground turmeric, ground ginger, ground cinnamon, and a pinch of ground black pepper to the saucepan. These spices have anti-inflammatory properties that can be beneficial for people with IBS.
- If desired, add a teaspoon of coconut oil to the mixture. Coconut oil can provide a creamy texture and healthy fats.
- Stir the mixture continuously until the spices are well incorporated and the milk is warm. Avoid boiling.
- Take the saucepan off the heat and let the mixture cool down a bit.
- If you prefer a touch of sweetness, add a teaspoon of honey or maple syrup to the latte.
- For an extra layer of flavor, sprinkle a dash of ground cardamom and a pinch of cayenne pepper into the latte.
- Pour the golden milk turmeric latte into a mug and enjoy it warm.

NUTRITIONAL VALUE PER SERVING:

- Calories: Approximately 50-70 kcal (depending on milk and sweetener used)
- Carbohydrates: 4-6 g
- Fiber: 1 g
- Sugars: 2-4 g
- Protein: 1 g
- Fat: 3-4 g
- Sodium: 150 mg (may vary based on milk)
- Potassium: 200 mg (may vary based on milk)

HEALTH BENEFITS

- Turmeric: Curcumin, the active compound in turmeric, has anti-inflammatory properties that may help alleviate symptoms like abdominal pain and discomfort in people with IBS.
- Ginger: Ginger aids digestion and can help reduce nausea and bloating, common symptoms of IBS.
- Cinnamon: Cinnamon may help regulate blood sugar levels and provide mild anti-inflammatory effects.
- Black Pepper: Including black pepper in the recipe enhances the absorption of curcumin from turmeric.

- Coconut Oil: Healthy fats in coconut oil can support gut health and add creaminess to the latte.
- Cardamom: This spice adds a delightful flavor and may aid digestion.
- Cayenne Pepper: The small amount of cayenne pepper can provide a gentle heat and may stimulate digestion.

GREEN SMOOTHIE WITH SPINACH AND KIWI

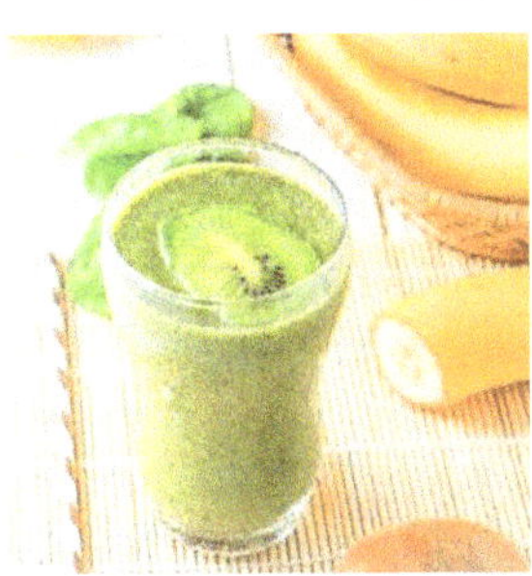

INGREDIENTS:

- 1 cup fresh spinach leaves (washed and stems removed)
- 2 ripe kiwis (peeled and chopped)
- 1 small banana (peeled and sliced)
- 1/2 cup unsweetened coconut water (or water)
- 1/2 cup unsweetened almond milk (or any preferred non-dairy milk)
- 1 tablespoon chia seeds (optional)
- 1/2 teaspoon freshly grated ginger
- Ice cubes

PROCEDURE:

- In a blender, add the fresh spinach leaves. Spinach is a low-FODMAP leafy green that's generally well-tolerated by many people with IBS.
- Add the peeled and chopped kiwis to the blender. Kiwis are rich in vitamins and fiber, which can support digestive health.
- Include the sliced banana for natural sweetness and creaminess. Choose a ripe banana for easier digestion.
- Pour in the unsweetened coconut water or water to help with blending and achieve the desired consistency.
- Add the unsweetened almond milk for added creaminess and nutrients. Almond milk is often well-tolerated by those with lactose sensitivity.

- If you prefer, include a tablespoon of chia seeds for added fiber and omega-3 fatty acids. Soak the chia seeds in liquid before blending for better digestion.
- Grate half a teaspoon of fresh ginger and add it to the blender. Ginger can help soothe digestive discomfort.
- Mix all the ingredients together until you get a creamy texture.
- If the smoothie is too thick, you can try adding a few ice cubes and blending it again.
- Pour the green smoothie into glasses and get it ready to be served.

NUTRITIONAL VALUE PER SERVING:

- Calories: Approximately 150-180 kcal
- Carbohydrates: 35-40 g
- Fiber: 8-10 g
- Sugars: 18-22 g
- Protein: 3-4 g
- Fat: 2-4 g
- Sodium: 100 mg (may vary based on ingredients)
- Potassium: 800 mg (may vary based on ingredients)

HEALTH BENEFITS

- Spinach: Spinach is rich in vitamins, minerals, and fiber, supporting healthy digestion and bowel regularity.
- Kiwi: Kiwi's natural enzymes can aid in digestion and its fiber content promotes gut health.
- Banana: A ripe banana offers gentle fiber, potassium, and natural sweetness that's easy on the stomach.
- Coconut Water: Hydrating and rich in electrolytes, coconut water can help maintain hydration levels, especially if diarrhea is a concern.
- Almond Milk: Almond milk is lactose-free and can provide a creamy texture without causing digestive issues.
- Chia Seeds: Chia seeds are a source of soluble fiber that can promote healthy digestion and may ease IBS symptoms.
- Ginger: Ginger's anti-inflammatory properties can help soothe gastrointestinal discomfort.

9

DESSERTS

CHIA SEED PUDDING WITH MIXED BERRIES

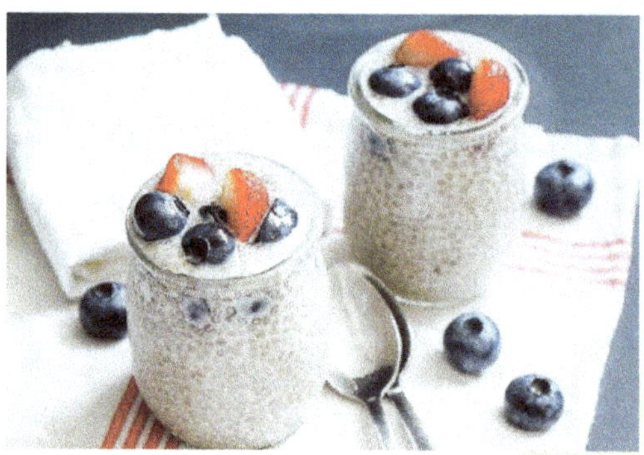

INGREDIENTS:

- 1/4 cup chia seeds
- One cup of almond milk (or any other non-dairy milk) is a great choice.
- 1 tablespoon maple syrup (optional)
- 1/2 teaspoon vanilla extract
- 1/2 cup mixed berries (blueberries, strawberries, raspberries)
- 1 tablespoon chopped nuts (almonds, walnuts) for garnish

PROCEDURE:

- In a bowl, combine chia seeds, almond milk, maple syrup (if using), and vanilla extract. Mix well to ensure that chia seeds are evenly distributed.
- Let the mixture sit for about 5-10 minutes, stirring occasionally.
- This enables the chia seeds to take in the liquid and form a pudding-like texture.
- After the initial rest, give the mixture one final stir and cover the bowl with plastic wrap or a lid.
- Put the mixture in the fridge for a minimum of two hours or let it sit overnight. This will give the chia seeds enough time to swell and thicken the mixture.
- When the pudding has set, give it a good stir to break up any clumps. If the pudding seems too thick, you can add a splash of almond milk to reach your desired consistency.
- Wash and prepare the mixed berries by cutting larger berries into bite-sized pieces.
- To serve, spoon the chia seed pudding into serving bowls or glasses.Sprinkle the mixed berries and chopped nuts on top.
- Drizzle with a little extra maple syrup if desired for added sweetness.
- Enjoy your delicious and nutritious Chia Seed Pudding with Mixed Berries!

NUTRITIONAL VALUE (PER SERVING):

- Calories: ~220 kcal
- Total Fat: 10g

- Saturated Fat: 1g
- Carbohydrates: 25g
- Dietary Fiber: 12g
- Sugars: 8g
- Protein: 6g

HEALTH BENEFITS

- Chia seeds are a great source of soluble fiber, which can help regulate bowel movements and alleviate constipation often experienced by people with IBS.
- Almond milk is low in FODMAPs (Fermentable Oligosaccharides, Disaccharides, Monosaccharides, and Polyols), making it a suitable dairy alternative for individuals following the low FODMAP diet.
- Mixed berries are rich in antioxidants and vitamins, which can contribute to gut health and provide essential nutrients while being gentle on the digestive system.
- This pudding is naturally gluten-free and contains no artificial additives, making it easy on the stomach for those with sensitivities.
- The optional use of maple syrup allows for customization of sweetness, catering to individual preferences and avoiding triggers.
- Nuts provide healthy fats and additional fiber, promoting satiety and potentially reducing inflammation.

BAKED APPLES WITH CINNAMON AND WALNUTS

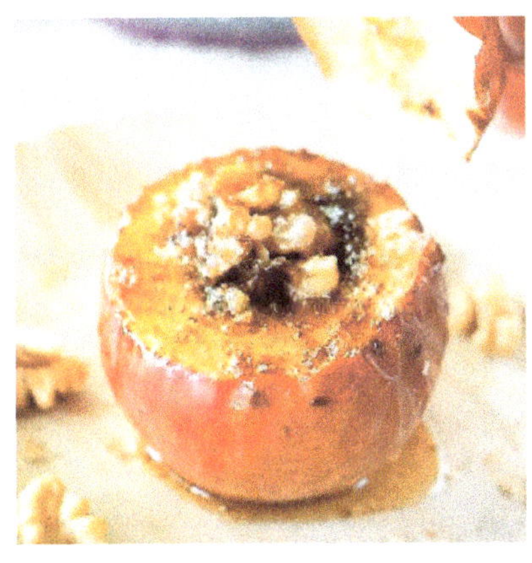

INGREDIENTS:

- 2 medium-sized apples (choose low-FODMAP varieties like Gala or Fuji)
- 2 tablespoons chopped walnuts

- 1 teaspoon ground cinnamon
- 1 tablespoon maple syrup (optional)
- 1 tablespoon coconut oil or lactose-free butter
- A pinch of salt

PROCEDURE:

- Preheat your oven to 350°F (175°C).
- Clean the apples carefully and pat them dry.
- Core the apples using an apple corer or a small knife, leaving the bottoms intact. This will create a well in the center for the filling.
- In a small bowl, mix the chopped walnuts, ground cinnamon, and a pinch of salt.
- Stuff each apple with the walnut-cinnamon mixture, pressing down gently to pack the filling.
- Put the apples filled with stuffing in a baking pan.
- If using maple syrup, drizzle a little over each apple.
- Place a small amount of coconut oil or lactose-free butter on top of each stuffed apple.
- Cover the baking dish with aluminum foil.
- Bake in the preheated oven for about 25-30 minutes or until the apples are tender but not mushy. Cooking time may vary based on the apple variety and size.
- Once baked, remove the foil and let the apples cool slightly before serving.
- Serve the baked apples warm, optionally with a dollop of lactose-free yogurt or a sprinkle of additional cinnamon.

NUTRITIONAL VALUE (PER SERVING):

- Calories: ~200 kcal
- Total Fat: 10g
- Saturated Fat: 3g
- Carbohydrates: 30g
- Dietary Fiber: 6g
- Sugars: 18g
- Protein: 2g

HEALTH BENEFITS

- Low-FODMAP apples are gentle on the digestive system and can provide essential vitamins and fiber without triggering IBS symptoms.
- Walnuts offer healthy fats and provide a source of omega-3 fatty acids, which have anti-inflammatory properties and can support gut health.

- Cinnamon may help reduce bloating and gas, common symptoms in people with IBS, and also adds a comforting flavor to the dish.
- Maple syrup (used in moderation) is a natural sweetener that's generally well-tolerated on the low-FODMAP diet. It adds a touch of sweetness without causing digestive discomfort.
- Coconut oil or lactose-free butter provide a source of healthy fats that are less likely to irritate the gut.
- The fiber content from the apples and walnuts can promote regular bowel movements and ease constipation, a common concern for individuals with IBS.

DARK CHOCOLATE AVOCADO MOUSSE

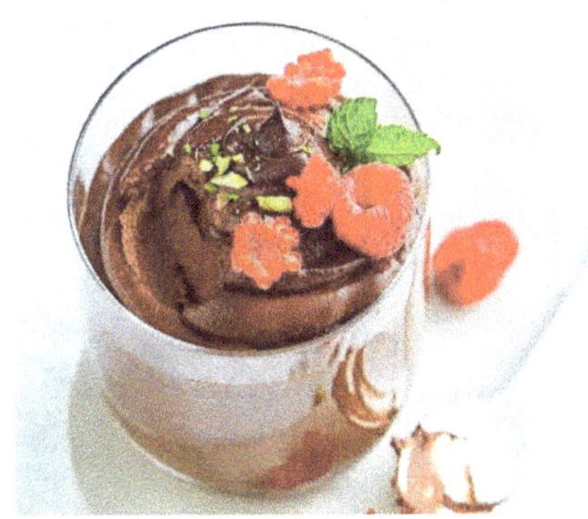

INGREDIENTS:

- 2 ripe avocados
- 1/4 cup dark cocoa powder (unsweetened)
- 1/4 cup maple syrup (or another low-FODMAP sweetener)
- 1 teaspoon vanilla extract
- A pinch of salt
- Optional toppings: chopped strawberries, sliced almonds

PROCEDURE:

- Divide the avocados in two, take out the stones, and scoop out the insides.
- Put the avocado meat into a food processor or blender.
- Add the dark cocoa powder, maple syrup, vanilla extract, and a pinch of salt to the avocados.
- Blend the ingredients until smooth and creamy.
- You may need to pause and scrape the sides of the blender or processor to make sure everything is blended properly.
- Taste the mousse and adjust sweetness or cocoa levels if desired.

- Once the mixture is smooth, spoon it into serving glasses or bowls.
- If desired, top the mousse with chopped strawberries and sliced almonds for extra flavor and texture.
- Refrigerate the mousse for at least 30 minutes before serving to allow it to chill and firm up.
- Enjoy the delicious and rich Dark Chocolate Avocado Mousse!

NUTRITIONAL VALUE (PER SERVING):

- Calories: ~180 kcal
- Total Fat: 14g
- Saturated Fat: 2g
- Carbohydrates: 18g
- Dietary Fiber: 7g
- Sugars: 9g
- Protein: 3g

HEALTH BENEFITS

- Avocado provides healthy fats and is low in FODMAPs, making it a great ingredient for those following an IBS elimination diet.
- Dark cocoa powder is a rich source of antioxidants and can potentially improve gut health by reducing inflammation.
- Maple syrup (or low-FODMAP sweetener) adds sweetness without causing digestive distress.
- This mousse is dairy-free, avoiding potential triggers for individuals with lactose intolerance or sensitivity.
- The high fiber content from avocados can promote regular bowel movements and alleviate symptoms of constipation often experienced by individuals with IBS.
- The monounsaturated fats from avocados can contribute to a healthy gut lining and reduce inflammation in the digestive tract.

10

MEAL PLANS

ONE-WEEK MEAL PLAN

DAY 1:

- Breakfast: Banana and cinnamon-sprinkled quinoa porridge.
- Lunch: Grilled chicken salad with mixed greens, carrots, and a simple olive oil and lemon dressing.
- Snack: Rice cakes with almond butter.
- Dinner: Baked salmon with steamed spinach and roasted sweet potatoes.

DAY 2:

- Breakfast: Greek yogurt topped with fruit and honey.
- Lunch: Turkey and avocado wrap with lettuce in a gluten-free wrap.
- Snack: Carrot and cucumber sticks with hummus.
- Dinner: Stir-fried tofu with bell peppers, zucchini, and brown rice.

DAY 3:

- Breakfast: spinach, tomatoes, and feta cheese in an omelet.
- Lunch: Quinoa and black bean bowl with salsa and a dollop of plain yogurt.
- Snack: Handful of mixed nuts.
- Dinner: Grilled shrimp with asparagus and quinoa.

DAY 4:

- Breakfast: Smoothie with spinach, pineapple, ginger, and coconut water.
- Lunch: Spinach and arugula salad with grilled chicken, strawberries, and a balsamic vinaigrette.
- Snack: Rice cakes with mashed avocado.
- Dinner: Baked cod with steamed broccoli and mashed potatoes.

DAY 5:

- Breakfast: Chia seed pudding with kiwi and slivered almonds.
- Lunch: lentil soup and gluten-free bread on the side.

- Snack: Rice crackers with tuna salad.
- Dinner:quinoa and grilled steak with roasted Brussels sprouts.

DAY 6:

- Breakfast: Brown rice cake topped with cottage cheese and sliced peaches.
- Lunch: Sushi bowl with cucumber, avocado, smoked salmon, and seaweed.
- Snack: Sliced bell peppers with guacamole.
- Dinner: Baked chicken with sautéed green beans and wild rice.

DAY 7:

- Breakfast: Overnight oats made with oats, almond milk, chia seeds, and topped with raspberries.
- Lunch: Roasted vegetable and quinoa salad with lemon-tahini dressing.
- Snack: Mixed berries and a handful of walnuts.
- Dinner: Marinara sauce with zucchini noodles with turkey meatballs.

TWO-WEEK REINTRODUCTION PHASE MEAL PLAN
WEEK 1:

DAY 1 - FRUCTANS REINTRODUCTION:

- Breakfast: spinach-topped scrambled eggs on gluten-free bread.
- Lunch: Grilled chicken salad with mixed greens, tomatoes, and a simple olive oil and balsamic vinegar dressing.
- Snack: Carrot sticks with lactose-free yogurt dip.
- Dinner: Quinoa bowl with sautéed zucchini, grilled steak, and a small amount of garlic-infused oil.

DAY 2 - SORBITOL REINTRODUCTION:

- Breakfast: Smoothie with banana, spinach, almond milk, and a touch of honey.
- Lunch: Turkey and avocado wrap with lettuce in a gluten-free wrap.
- Snack: Rice cakes with almond butter.
- Dinner: Grilled chicken with steamed green beans and mashed sweet potatoes.

DAY 3 - FRUCTOSE REINTRODUCTION:

- Breakfast: Oatmeal with strawberries and a drizzle of maple syrup.
- Lunch: Tuna salad with mixed greens, cucumbers, and a lemon-tahini dressing.
- Snack: Mixed berries.
- Dinner: Baked salmon with roasted carrots and quinoa.

DAY 4 - MANNITOL REINTRODUCTION:

- Breakfast: Greek yogurt with kiwi and a sprinkle of chia seeds.
- Lunch: Lentil soup with a side of gluten-free bread.
- Snack: avocado mashed with rice cakes.
- Dinner: Stir-fried tofu with bell peppers, broccoli, and brown rice.

WEEK 2:

DAY 5 - GOS REINTRODUCTION:

- Breakfast: Chia seed pudding with pineapple and slivered almonds.
- Lunch: Sushi bowl with cucumber, avocado, smoked salmon, and seaweed.
- Snack: Mixed nuts.
- Dinner: Baked cod with sautéed spinach and wild rice.

DAY 6 - LACTOSE REINTRODUCTION:

- Breakfast: Overnight oats made with oats, lactose-free milk, and blueberries.
- Lunch: Spinach and arugula salad with grilled chicken, strawberries, and a balsamic vinaigrette.
- Snack: Lactose-free yogurt with raspberries.
- Dinner: Grilled steak with roasted Brussels sprouts and mashed potatoes made with lactose-free milk.

DAY 7 - REPEAT AND OBSERVE:

- Choose one of the FODMAP groups you reintroduced and include foods from that group in your meals throughout the day.
- Keep an eye out for any symptoms or responses.

DAY 8-14 - OBSERVE AND PLAN:

- Continue observing how your body reacts to the reintroduced FODMAP groups.
- Pay attention to any signs or uneasiness you may be feeling.
- Based on your observations, you can then decide which FODMAP groups you can tolerate and in what quantities. Remember, this is a general sample meal plan and should be customized to your preferences and needs.

CONCLUSION

The IBS Elimination Diet Cookbook offers not just a collection of recipes, but a journey towards improved well-being and a happier digestive system. This cookbook empowers you to take charge of your health by providing delicious, nourishing meals carefully crafted to support the elimination phase of the FODMAP diet. With its vibrant array of flavors and thoughtfully curated dishes, this cookbook is your reliable companion on the path to discovering trigger foods, soothing discomfort, and embracing a more fulfilling lifestyle.

Let this cookbook be your culinary guide, offering not only a variety of scrumptious recipes but also a sense of community and understanding. As you embark on this journey, remember that each meal is a step towards reclaiming your comfort and vitality. With determination, creativity, and the guidance of the IBS Elimination Diet Cookbook, you're equipped to cultivate a happier, healthier relationship with food. Embrace the possibilities, savor the flavors, and revel in the positive changes that this cookbook can bring to your life. Your digestive wellness matters, and this cookbook is here to celebrate your commitment to it.

www.ingramcontent.com/pod-product-compliance
Lightning Source LLC
Chambersburg PA
CBHW080940260726
48661CB00010B/4010